BONE *Vivant!*

Calcium-Enhanced Recipes and Bone-Building Exercises

BONE *Vivant!*

Calcium-Enhanced Recipes and Bone-Building Exercises

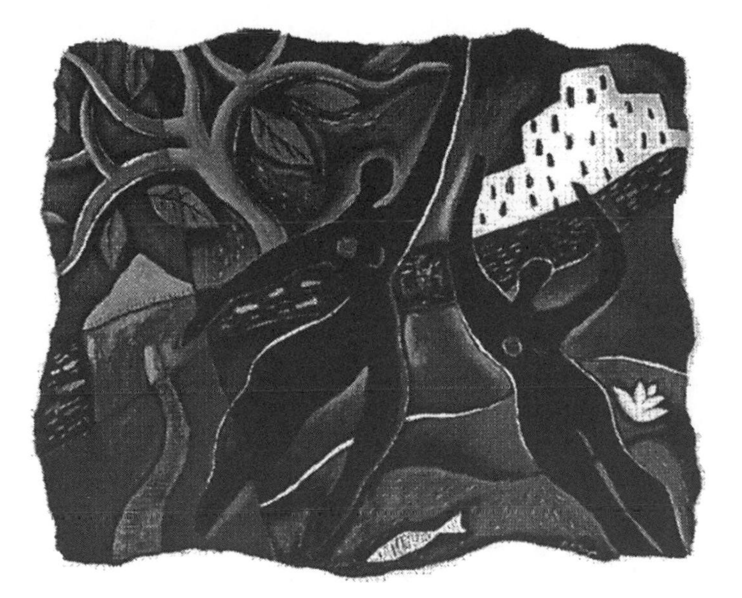

JAN MAIN *in co-operation with*
THE OSTEOPOROSIS SOCIETY OF CANADA

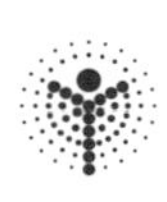

Macmillan Canada
Toronto

Canadian Cataloguing in Publication Data

Main, Jan

Bone vivant! : calcium-enhanced recipes and bone-building exercises

Includes index.

ISBN 0-7715-7455-X

1. High-calcium diet – Recipes. 2. Osteoporosis – Exercise therapy. 3. Osteoporosis – Prevention. I. Title.

RM237.56.M34 1997 641.5'632 C97-930323-0

1 2 3 4 5 TRI 01 00 99 98 97

Cover and text design by Sharon Foster
Cover illustration by Helen d'Souza
Interior photographs by Douglas Bradshaw Photography
Illustrations by Bradley Kostynuik-freelancelot
Composition by IBEX Graphic Communications Inc.

Macmillan Canada wishes to thank the Canada Council, the Ontario Ministry of Culture and Communications and the Ontario Arts Council for supporting its publishing program. Macmillan Canada also wishes to thank the Osteoporosis Society of Canada for its support of *Bone Vivant!*

This book is available at special discounts for bulk purchases by your group or organization for sales promotions, premiums, fundraising and seminars. For details, contact: Macmillan Canada, Special Sales Department, 29 Birch Avenue, Toronto, ON M4V 1E2. Tel: 416-963-8830.

Macmillan Canada
A Division of Canada Publishing Corporation
Toronto, Ontario, Canada

To my dear friend Joan and my daughter, Alexa.
To mothers and daughters everywhere

Contents

Preface

One in four Canadian women over the age of 50 has osteoporosis and one in eight men over 50 also suffers from the disease. Another two million Canadians are at risk of developing osteoporosis as they reach their middle and senior years.

Osteoporosis is characterized by low bone mass and deterioration of bone tissue. This in turn leads to fragile bones and risk of fracture. Fractures of the hip, wrist and vertebrae are most common. While most of us associate these fractures with falls, the unfortunate reality is that individuals with osteoporosis can fracture a bone even when doing such ordinary activities as picking up a child, being hugged or even sneezing.

While we don't know everything there is to know about osteoporosis, we do know many of the risk factors that contribute to an individual's chance of developing the disease. Women are more likely to develop osteoporosis than men, and post-menopausal women are at higher risk because they have lost the bone-building benefits of estrogen. Individuals of white or Eurasian ancestry are also at higher risk. Genetics play a strong role—if someone in our family has the disease, there is a greater chance we will develop it.

Lifestyle factors also play a strong role in osteoporosis. A calcium-rich diet and physical exercise are important not only to develop strong bones in our younger years, but to maintain bones as we age. It's never too late to improve our bone health.

This book recognizes that our lives are often a daily balancing act between families, friends, career and outside commitments. But eating a healthy diet and developing good exercise habits don't have to be hard work. *Bone Vivant!* provides recipes and nutrition hints that can help us increase our calcium intake while enjoying tasty meals; the exercise section provides easy exercises which can be incorporated into the daily activities of people of all ages.

Osteoporosis is a serious disease. But the good news is that each of us can take simple steps to reduce our risk of developing the disease or to slow its progression.

The Osteoporosis Society of Canada is committed to educating Canadians about osteoporosis and supporting individuals and communities in the prevention and treatment of the disease. We hope *Bone Vivant!* provides you with useful health information and a fresh repertoire of healthy meals. Happy cooking!

Roslyne Buchanan
President, Osteoporosis Society of Canada

Robert Josse, MD, FRCP(C)
Chair, Scientific Advisory Board
Osteoporosis Society of Canada
Professor of Medicine,
University of Toronto

Bone China Tea or Coffee Break? Your Choice!

When the weather turns bone-chilling damp and cold, and then the sidewalks turn icy, do you head for home and hearth? Why not invite your friends in to join you for a fundraising Bone China Tea this November, for Osteoporosis Month? Or if visiting your local café entices you more, then invite friends to relax with you over a steaming cup of calcium-rich caffe latte or mocaccino.

Osteoporosis is a crippling bone disease that strikes one in four women over 50 years of age. Tragically, diagnosis of this disease is too often by fracture—sometimes a break caused by a slip on the ice, sometimes a broken bone caused by a hug. Called the silent thief, osteoporosis robs bone of strength without much sign or warning.

Prevention starts with lifestyle habits established early. This is why we need your help. Together with your friends, your donations will assist the Osteoporosis Society of Canada (OSC) in expanding osteoporosis prevention education.

By hosting a Bone China Tea or a Coffee Break, you can:

- provide information so friends can protect themselves from the silent thief;
- share warm cheer;
- enjoy delicious delicacies that feature calcium by using recipes from *Bone Vivant!*;
- win prizes for your guests.

As host, you will receive a special gift from us. In addition, for $75 raised by the group, your guests may draw for a tea or coffee spoon; for $100 raised, a sampler with assorted teas or coffees; for $150, a copy of *Bone Vivant!*; and for $200, the draw winner will receive a designer cup that will become your guests' hot favorite.

To order your invitations, osteoporosis prevention information and tea or coffee guide, please call 1-800-463-6842. And thank you for your bone-warming support!

If you're wondering what to serve at your Bone China Tea, take a look at the photo opposite page 144 for some ideas. Try the Scones with Cheddar Cheese (p. 25), Chocolate Apricot Chews (p. 137), Molasses Crinkles (p. 138), Cranberry Orange Chutney (p. 43), Almond Shortbread (p. 136) or a spread made from the Savoury Cheddar and Orange Cheesecake (p. 51).

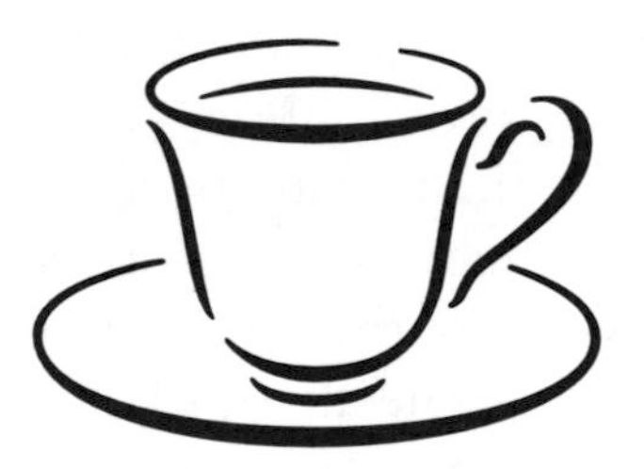

A MESSAGE FROM THE ONTARIO SOYBEAN GROWERS' MARKETING BOARD

Soybeans have been a dietary staple in Asian cultures for thousands of years. Tofu was first made in China around 200 B.C. and its popularity soon spread to Japan and neighbouring countries. Today, this delicate food is made fresh daily in thousands of small tofu shops throughout Asia. Only recently, however, have soyfoods made it on to North American plates. Their introduction is long overdue.

Soyfoods are a good source of many essential nutrients including protein, iron, fiber, calcium and B-vitamins. For example, 1 serving of soybeans (1/2 cup) contains approximately 14.3 g protein, 4.4 mg iron, 1.8 g fiber, 88 mg calcium and is a good source of some B-vitamins. The variety of soybean products is extensive. Tofu is probably the most well-known soyfood but whole soybeans, soy flour, textured soy protein, soy beverage, miso and tempeh are also available.

While the nutritional value of soyfoods is reason enough to add them to your diet, research into the broader health benefits of soy is on-going. Scientists are currently examining the role certain compounds in soybeans play in reducing the risk of cancer, heart disease and osteoporosis.

The Ontario Soybean Growers' Marketing Board recognizes the importance of diet in maintaining good health. For this reason, we are proud to sponsor *Bone Vivant!* Because osteoporosis may be prevented, it is vital that Canadians learn about this disease and take steps to avoid it. Exercise and a healthy diet, including soyfoods, are good ways to lower the risk of developing osteoporosis.

If you want to learn more about soybeans, please contact:

The Ontario Soybean Growers' Marketing Board
Box 1199, Chatham, Ontario, N7M 5L8

Phone: (519) 352-7730 Fax: (519)352-8983
E-mail: cansoy@ciaccess.com

Tom Lassaline
Chairman

Fred Brandenburg
Secretary-Manager

Author's Acknowledgments

I would like to extend my sincere thanks to a number of people whose help was invaluable:

To the wonderful group of professionals at the Osteoporosis Society whose enthusiasm and hard work made this project a pleasure, with special thanks to Mary Bowyer for attention to detail, Sue Berlove and the dedicated team of volunteers.

To Lesleigh Landry, professional chef and friend, for her organization, stamina and expertise in testing recipes.

To Barbara Selley at Info Access (1988) Inc., who provided much more than nutrient analysis and made herself available at all hours.

To the team of physiotherapists—Margaret Wells (Chair, Rehabilitation, Osteoporosis Society of Canada), Florinda Coelho (St. Joseph's Health Centre) and Josie Tominac (The Queen Elizabeth Hospital), for their assistance with the exercises.

To Dr. Susan Barr, University of British Columbia, School of Family and Nutritional Studies, and Heather McKay, University of British Columbia, School of Human Kinetics, for reviewing the material.

To Maureen McTeer, who conducted the five Bone China Teas across the country to prepare the way for *Bone Vivant!*

To the Macmillan staff and editor Susan Girvan, for their commitment to the endeavor.

To Richard and Susan Mackenzie of Toronto and Pat Hunt of Naismith Gloucester, who entered the "Name the Cookbook" contest and came up with *Bone Vivant!*

To Faye Clack Marketing and Communications, who allowed me to use the Sweet Potato Vichyssoise recipe.

ABOUT THE NUTRIENT INFORMATION ON THE RECIPES

Nutrient analysis of the recipes was performed by Info Access (1988) Inc., Don Mills, Ontario using the nutritional accounting component of the CBORD Menu Management System. The nutrient database was the 1991 Canadian Nutrient File supplemented with documented data from reliable sources. The analysis was based on imperial weights and measures, the smaller number of servings (i.e. larger portion) when there was a range, and the first ingredient listed when there was a choice. Optional ingredients and ingredients in unspecified amounts were not included.

Nutrient values have been rounded to the nearest whole number; non-zero values less than 0.5 are shown as "trace."

HEALTHY NUTRIENT INTAKES

Calcium and Vitamin D

The Osteoporosis Society of Canada's current recommended intakes for calcium and vitamin D can be found on pages 4 and 8. In some cases, the amounts recommended are higher than the Recommended Daily Intakes upon which Canadian nutrition labelling is based.

Calories, Protein, Fat and Carbohydrate

Health Canada recommends the following daily intakes of Calories (energy), protein, fat and carbohydrate.

Recommended Nutrient Intakes

	Women		Men	
Age	25–49	50–74	25–49	50–74
Calories	1900	1800	2700	2300
Protein	51g	54 g	64 g	63 g
Fat (up to 30% of Calories)	63 g	60 g	90 g	77 g
Carbohydrate (55% of Calories or more)	260 g	250 g	370 g	315 g

Dietary Fiber

An intake of at least 20 grams per day is a common recommendation. Amounts greatly in excess of this level, however, may hinder absorption of calcium and other minerals.

Sodium

Health Canada recommends that we reduce our sodium intake (typically 3500 to 4600 mg per day in industrialized countries) by minimizing salt used in cooking and at the table and by cutting down on commercial foods containing salt and other sodium compounds. As a guideline, remember that one-quarter teaspoon (1 mL) salt contains approximately 600 mg sodium.

Magnesium

Magnesium, a mineral required for healthy bones, is widely distributed in fruits and vegetables, whole-grain products, dairy products, meat and nuts. Recommended daily intakes for women are 200 mg for 25 to 49 years and 210 mg for 50 to 74 years; recommended intake for men 25 to 74 years is 250 mg.

READING FOOD LABELS

Nutrition panels on packaged foods report minerals and vitamins as percentages of the Recommended Daily Intakes established for nutrition labelling (*Guide to Food Labelling and Advertising*, 1996, Agriculture and Agri-Food Canada). Refer to the following chart to convert label quantities of calcium and magnesium to milligrams (mg), and vitamin D to International Units (IU).

Nutrient	100% Recommended Daily Intake for Labelling (RDI)
Calcium	1100 mg
Magnesium	250 mg
Vitamin D	200 IU

Example:

25% RDI of vitamin D = .25 x 200 IU = 50 IU

Introduction

Bone Vivant! is a workbook to promote a lifetime of healthy, living bone. Yes, our bones are living. They are largely made up of the essential mineral calcium and are constantly breaking down and being built up again. This renewal process is called **bone remodelling**. Up until about age 35, the "building up" phase exceeds or is matched by the "breaking down" phase, meaning that, for the body as a whole, bone is maintained. After this age, the repair process slows down in both men and women and bone can be lost.

Calcium is required not only by bone, but also by every cell in the body for proper functioning. We cannot manufacture calcium; therefore, we must get it from our diets. If our diet does not give us enough calcium, then the body's regulatory system will take calcium from our bones to maintain the necessary level in our blood for use by other tissues. The goal of good calcium nutrition is to keep a balance of calcium where our calcium loss does not exceed our dietary intake; otherwise, the body will dip into the bone store for necessary calcium.

In childhood, calcium is necessary to grow a healthy skeleton. By age 15 to 20, the bones stop growing in length. In early adulthood, somewhere between ages 20 to 30, calcium, combined with regular physical activity and normal hormonal status, strengthens the bone, helping us put a supply of calcium in our bones to maintain their strength. This is referred to as reaching **peak bone mass**. The greater this peak bone mass, the less likely our bones are to become porous and fragile as we age. If bones become so fragile and brittle they break easily, the condition is called **osteoporosis**. This debilitating disease can result in bones so fragile that even a sneeze can cause a fracture.

Osteoporosis is appropriately called the "silent thief." It silently robs the bones of calcium without any symptoms until a fracture occurs. By that time, the damage is done. Although osteoporosis can be treated, it is far better to prevent the disease from occurring. Prevention starts in childhood. Prevention is the goal of *Bone Vivant!*

There are many factors related to osteoporosis prevention. The two which we can most strongly influence ourselves are:

- **a balanced calcium-rich diet**
- **regular activity**

Calcium is important for building strong bones in childhood, maintaining bone density in adults and reducing the likelihood of fractures as we age.

Activity, especially weight-bearing activity, is important for healthy bones because bones need the stress of activity to help build and maintain strong bones. For example, if we are immobile—perhaps confined to bed—we lose bone.

WHO IS AT RISK OF GETTING OSTEOPOROSIS?

Osteoporosis affects one in four women over 50 and one in eight men over 50. A total of 1.4 million Canadians have osteoporosis, and another two million women and men are at risk of developing the disease.

Some people are more likely to develop the condition than others.

Below is a list of known risk factors that predispose you to develop osteoporosis. If you have four or more risk factors from this list, check with your doctor concerning your risk and the possibility of having your bone density measured. (See Diagnosing the Disease, p. 4) Although these are the risk factors associated with the disease, there is still much to learn about osteoporosis. In some cases, individuals develop osteoporosis without these risk factors.

Risk Factors

- female
- prolonged hormonal imbalance, i.e. have stopped menstruating for a period of time because of eating disorders, stress or excessive exercise
- past menopause—either natural or induced. Risk is greater if menopause occurs before age 45
- age 50 or older for both men and women
- insufficient calcium in the diet
- insufficient vitamin D
- insufficient physical activity
- family history of osteoporosis
- thin, small-boned body frame
- white or Eurasian background
- smoker
- caffeine consumption—more than 3 cups daily of tea, coffee or cola
- alcohol consumption, consistently more than 2 drinks a day
- prolonged or excessive use of certain medications—cortisone, prednisone, thyroid hormone, anticonvulsants and antacids containing aluminum

Hormones and Calcium Balance

The female hormones estrogen and progesterone also play an important part in slowing down bone loss and reducing the chances of breaking bones. At the time of menopause, women stop producing these hormones, leaving our bones vulnerable. Making the decision whether to take hormone therapy can be difficult. You may wish to talk to your physician as well as any of your friends who've had to make this decision.

Controlling the Risk Factors

While some risk factors are beyond our control, we can take positive steps to modify others. We can control:

- our calcium intake

- our vitamin D intake
- how much exercise we do
- how much caffeine we consume
- whether or not we smoke
- how much alcohol we consume
- to some extent, the medication and hormones we use (check with your doctor)

DIAGNOSING THE DISEASE

Bone Vivant! is all about prevention. However if you have four or more risk factors, discuss this with your doctor who may request a bone densitometry test. Bone densitometry measures the amount of bone in the lower spine or hip to determine your risk of fracture. This test is similar to an X-ray although a standard X-ray will not show osteoporosis until you have lost at least one quarter of your bone density. Bone density tests are not available everywhere. In this case, it is even more important to know the risk factors and take preventative measures.

GETTING ENOUGH CALCIUM

How much is enough?

The Osteoporosis Society recommends the following amounts of calcium every day to maintain strong bones, preserve bone mass and reduce the risk of fracture.

Age	Recommended Daily Intake
7 to 9	700 mg
10 to 12 (boys)	900 mg
10 to 12 (girls)[1]	1,200–1,400 mg
13 to 16	1,200–1,400 mg
17 to 18	1,200 mg
19 to 49	1,000 mg
50+	1,000–1,500 mg[2]

[1] On average girls go through their adolescent growth spurt two years earlier than boys and require more calcium for this growth spurt.

[2] A minimum of 1,000 mg is recommended but higher intakes may be advisable if the risk of osteoporosis is high.

Calcium and Life Cycle

- Calcium needs are high during the **growth** spurts of children, particularly the teen years when bones are growing in length.

- Calcium needs are high during adult years to **maintain** bone mass and because calcium is not as well absorbed as in childhood.
- Calcium needs increase after age 50: in women because of the loss of the hormone **estrogen** which protects the body from bone loss; and also due to the reduced ability of older men and women to **absorb** calcium from the diet.

Where do we get calcium?

The best place to get calcium is from the food we eat. To determine if you are getting enough calcium, consult the chart below and estimate your daily intake of calcium, and compare it to the recommended amounts indicated in the previous chart. If you fall short of the recommended amount, plan on ways of improving your calcium intake. If this proves difficult for some reason, then consider a calcium supplement.

Approximate Calcium Content of Some Common Foods

	Portion	Calcium (mg)
MILK, MILK PRODUCTS, MILK SUBSTITUTE		
Milk (skim, 1%, 2%, homogenized)	1 cup/250 mL	300
Buttermilk and chocolate milk	1 cup/250 mL	285
Soy beverage	1 cup/250 mL	10
Evaporated milk, undiluted	1/2 cup/125 mL	350
Instant skim milk powder	3 tbsp/50 mL	155
Ice cream	1/2 cup/125 mL	80
Light sour cream	1 tbsp/50 mL	30
Sour cream	1 tbsp/50 mL	15
Plain yogurt	175 g/3/4 cup	300
Fruit yogurt	175 g/3/4 cup	250
Swiss cheese (1″ x 1″ x 3″/ 2.5 cm x 2.5 cm x 7.5 cm)	1 3/4 oz/50 g	480
Light Cheddar cheese (1″ x 1″ x 3″/ 2.5 cm x 2.5 cm x 7.5 cm)	1 3/4 oz/50 g	385
Cheddar cheese	1 3/4 oz/50 g	360
Grated Parmesan cheese	1 tbsp/15 mL	85
Cream cheese	1 tbsp/15 mL	12
Ricotta cheese	1/2 cup/125 ml	255
Light ricotta cheese	1/2 cup/125 ml	335
Cottage cheese	1/2 cup/125 mL	75

	Portion	Calcium (mg)
MEAT, FISH, POULTRY, ALTERNATIVES		
Salmon including bones, canned, drained	Half 213 g/7½ oz can	225
Sardines, including bones, 8 small, drained	45 g/1½ oz	165
Tuna, canned, drained	Half 213 g/7½ oz can	23
Turkey, dark meat, roasted, no skin	90 g 3 oz	27
Turkey, light meat, roasted, no skin	90 g/3 oz	16
Chicken, light or dark meat, roasted, no skin	90 g/3 oz	13
Egg	1 large	24
Pork, roasted, lean only	90 g/3 oz	24
Lamb, roasted, lean only,	90 g/3 oz	12
Beef, roasted, lean only	90 g/3 oz	8
SHELLFISH		
Clams, canned, drained	½ cup/125 mL	75
Shrimp, canned, drained	½ cup/125 mL	40
Crab, canned drained	½ cup/125 mL	28
Mussels, cooked	2 medium	25
Oysters, raw	2 medium	10
LEGUMES AND TOFU		
Soybeans, canned or boiled	1 cup/250 mL	175
Baked beans, canned or boiled	1 cup/250 mL	150
Navy beans, canned or boiled	1 cup/250 mL	125
Pinto beans, canned or boiled	1 cup/250 mL	85
Chick-peas, canned or boiled	1 cup/250 mL	75
Kidney beans, canned or boiled	1 cup/250 mL	55
Tofu, containing 10 percent of Recommended Daily Intake of calcium per 90 g*	½ cup/250 mL cubed 3 oz/90 g	110
NUTS AND SEEDS		
Almonds	½ cup/250 mL	190
Hazelnuts	½ cup/250 mL	130
Sesame seeds	½ cup/250 mL	100
Walnuts	½ cup/250 mL	45
Pecans	½ cup/250 mL	20
BAKING INGREDIENTS		
Soy flour	1 cup/250 mL	240
All purpose flour	1 cup/250 mL	20
Blackstrap molasses	2 tbsp/25 mL	280
Fancy molasses	2 tbsp/25 mL	70
PASTA (weight and measure before cooking)		
Soy pasta (e.g. ¾ cup macaroni)	85 g/3 oz	24
Regular pasta (e.g. ¾ cup macaroni)	85 g/3 oz	16

Item	Portion	Calcium (mg)
BREAD		
White bread	1 slice	20
Whole wheat bread	1 slice	24
FRUIT		
Figs, dried, chopped	½ cup/250 mL	120
Currants, dried, chopped	½ cup/250 mL	60
Raisins	½ cup/250 mL	40
Apricots, dried, chopped	½ cup/250 mL	30
Dates, dried, chopped	½ cup/250 mL	30
Oranges, whole, fresh	1 medium	50
VEGETABLES**		
Bok-choy, shredded, raw	½ cup/125 mL	35
Bok-choy, shredded, cooked	½ cup/125 mL	80
Broccoli, chopped, raw	½ cup/125 mL	20
Broccoli, chopped, cooked	½ cup/125 mL	35
Cabbage, shredded, raw	½ cup/125 mL	15
Cabbage, shredded, cooked	½ cup/125 mL	25
Collards, chopped, cooked	½ cup/125 mL	15
Kale, chopped, raw	½ cup/125 mL	45
Mustard greens, chopped, cooked	½ cup/125 mL	52
Nappa, shredded, raw	½ cup/125 mL	30
Turnip greens, chopped, raw	½ cup/125 mL	105

*On labels, calcium content is expressed as a percentage of Recommended Daily Intake (%RDI). To determine calcium content in mg, multiply %RDI by 1100. E.g., 15% RDI = 15% x 1100 = 165 mg.

**A volume of cooked vegetables (e.g., ½ cup/125 mL) will have a higher calcium content than the same quantity of raw; the change in texture resulting from cooking means more vegetable can be packed in.

Absorption of Calcium

1. A daily **well-balanced diet** including foods rich in calcium is the best way to ensure absorbing the calcium you eat to produce healthy bones. The foods that can be well absorbed are listed in the chart showing calcium content. Milk and dairy products are excellent sources of calcium because they are rich in calcium and they are well absorbed. Many people find it difficult to get enough calcium without including milk or milk products in their diet.

2. **Bio-availability:** Bio-availability refers to the **availability** of the nutrient to our bodies, i.e. how well it can be absorbed. There are some vegetables that contain calcium, but they also contain *oxalates* which bind with the calcium making it unavailable to the body. Thus, this calcium is not bio-available. These foods are spinach, rhubarb and beet greens. Although they are nutritious foods, they cannot be considered a source of calcium.

   Likewise, many high fiber foods such as cereals, legumes and vegetables contain *phytates* which bind with the calcium, hindering the absorption of calcium. Vegetables containing oxalates and grains containing phytates are still nutritious foods contributing other essential nutrients but they cannot be considered a source of calcium.
3. **Vitamin D** is critical for calcium absorption. Vitamin D is made by our bodies by the action of sun on the skin. Provided we are exposed to sun for 15 minutes a day on our hands and face, we should be getting sufficient sunlight to make the necessary vitamin D. However, in northern climates, there is insufficient sun from October to March. Some people may be housebound or may be using sunscreen, making it impossible for them to get the necessary exposure to sunlight. These individuals need to get vitamin D from other sources. Health Canada's current recommended level for vitamin D is 100 IU for adults up to 49 and 200 IU in adults aged 50 and older. The Osteoporosis Society recommends that adults receive 400 IU per day. Older adults and those with osteoporosis need an intake of 400 to 800 IU per day.

   How can we get vitamin D? Milk and margarine are fortified with vitamin D. Each cup (250 mL) of milk contains 100 IU while one tablespoon (15 mL) of margarine has 80 IU. If you are following a calcium-rich diet including milk you should have enough vitamin D. Other sources of vitamin D are salmon, sardines, herring, mackerel, swordfish and fish liver oils from halibut and cod. If you are not exposed to sunlight or do not drink milk on a regular basis or do not eat the foods listed above in sufficient quantity, the Osteoporosis Society recommends that you may need a multi-vitamin supplement which contains 400 IU of vitamin D. Before taking a supplement, check with your doctor as excessive vitamin D can be harmful.

Vitamin D Content (Approximate) of Some Common Foods

	Portion	Vitamin D (IU)
Milk (skim, 1%, 2% homogenized, chocolate)	1 cup/250 mL	100
Buttermilk	1 cup/250 mL	0
Soy beverage	1 cup/250 mL	0
Evaporated milk, undiluted	1/2 cup/125 mL	110
Margarine	1 tsp/5 mL	25
Salmon, canned, drained	Half 213 g/7 1/2 oz can	700
Sardines, 8 small, drained	45 g/1 1/2 oz	75

Calcium Loss Through the Urine

1. **Too much protein** in our diet can increase the amount of calcium lost in the urine. Eat the amounts of meat or alternatives outlined in Canada's Food Guide to Healthy Eating, two or three servings a day. For example, one serving is 2 to 3 oz of meat, fish or poultry, 1 or 2 eggs or 1/3 cup (75 mL) tofu.
2. **Too much salt** in our diet increases the loss of calcium in the urine. Most processed food we eat contains salt so we should avoid adding more salt to season food. Processed foods containing salt are: salty snack foods such as potato chips; processed meats such as luncheon meats; commercial soups and sauces; crackers; commercial cookies; frozen, pre-made dinners; commercial salad dressings; packaged pasta dinners with sauce mixes; pickles and relishes.
3. **Too much caffeine** increases calcium loss through the urine. Caffeine is contained in coffee, chocolate, tea and cola beverages. Coffee has more

Salt Tips:
Although processed foods are a convenience, wherever possible, try making your own soups, sauces, dressings and pasta sauces. This way you control the ingredients you use and can control the amount of salt included in a dish.

caffeine than tea. Two or three cups of coffee a day is considered safe providing you are following a diet with the recommended levels of calcium.

Caffeine Content of Common Foods

	Quantity	Caffeine (mg)
Chocolate, bitter, baking	1 oz	14
Chocolate, milk, plain	1 oz	6
Cocoa	2 tbsp	24
Coffee, brewed	3/4 cup	103
Coffee, instant	3/4 cup	57
Coffee, instant, decaffeinated	3/4 cup	2
Cola, carbonated beverage	355 mL	37
Cola, carbonated beverage with Aspartame	355 mL	50
Tea, brewed	3/4 cup	35

Can You Get Too Much Calcium?

It used to be thought that if you had too much calcium in your diet you could increase your risk of kidney stones. Most experts now agree that calcium consumption does not affect the development of kidney stones, especially if the calcium is derived from food.

Caffeine Tips:

- **If you like a full-flavored coffee, opt for a dark roast like espresso which actually has less caffeine.**
- **It is a good idea to have a cup of milk for every additional cup of coffee over the recommended 3-cup limit.**
- **Try café au lait where there is a good deal of milk incorporated with the coffee.**
- **Use decaffeinated coffee.**
- **Steep tea no more than 3 minutes to minimize the caffeine in the brew.**

LACTOSE INTOLERANCE

If you are lactose intolerant, that is, you cannot digest the sugars in milk, you may find it difficult to include milk in your diet. *The Lactose-Free Family Cookbook* (Jan Main, Macmillan Canada, 1996) deals with this topic and has a number of recipes, both vegetarian and non-vegetarian, that you may find helpful. Here are some suggestions to assist you with this condition:

- try lactose-reduced milk.
- try milk in small quantities, about 1/4 cup (50 mL) at a time.
- use only hard, aged cheese like Parmesan or aged Cheddar. Start with small quantities and work up to the quantity you can tolerate.

- yogurt may be tolerated because it contains bacteria which breaks down the milk sugar, lactose.
- try small amounts of chocolate milk or whole milk which are digested more slowly.
- try lactase drops or pills which digest the lactose in your system.
- if you are too sensitive for any milk product, then incorporate the other calcium-rich foods from the chart on page 5 in your diet and consult a doctor about taking a calcium supplement. If you are unable to consume milk or dairy products, you are probably only getting about 300 mg of calcium per day.
- incorporate tofu coagulated with calcium chloride or calcium sulfate in your diet as an alternative calcium source. For more information on tofu, see below.

TOFU

Tofu, also called soybean curd, is the vegetarian equivalent of cottage cheese in the dairy world. It is made by combining fresh, hot soy beverage with a coagulant to cause curdling. Tofu may be a calcium source if the coagulant used is either calcium chloride or calcium sulfate. You must read the ingredient list on the side of the package to determine whether calcium chloride or calcium sulfate is present (see footnote to calcium content chart on p. 7). Tofu is a calcium source especially useful for a vegan diet which does not include milk, milk products or fish.

Check the package for the expiry date as well as the coagulant used. Like a dairy food, tofu has a shelf life and must be used before the expiry date. Buy it from a refrigerated counter and keep it refrigerated.

There are two types of tofu: silken and cotton. It will be marked silken on the package. If unmarked, assume it is cotton. This refers to the method used to make the tofu. If it is silken, it will have a smooth, custard-like texture; the texture will be slightly coarser if it is cotton. Both types of tofu need to be drained before using. In the case of cotton tofu, drain it and cover with fresh water daily until you're ready to use it.

There are also three different consistencies of tofu: soft, firm and extra firm. Use the type and consistency specified in the recipe. Generally, soft tofu is used in drinks, spreads and dips. I recommend silken soft tofu for dips and spreads to replace cream cheese and sour cream. Firm tofu is used in stews, soups and cheesecakes, while extra firm can be grilled or stir-fried.

Tofu is bland and requires extra herbs and seasoning for flavor. Spicy mixtures, like chili and Caesar Dressing (p. 91) are a great way of incorporating this calcium-rich food into your diet. For more recipe ideas, consult *The Lactose-Free Family Cookbook*.

Chapter 1

Morning Starts

You need good sources of calcium all day long. You can start at breakfast with milk on your cereal or get an extra dose of calcium-rich milk by using it instead of water to make porridge. No time for breakfast, you say? What about a hot, brimming cup of café au lait or a cool, refreshing fruit shake on the run? Another way to get some calcium is to pick up a bagel with Cheddar cheese on your way to work.

Don't forget the orange. Generally, when people think about the nutritional value of oranges, vitamin C comes to mind. However, this fruit also contains valuable calcium. Next time you are rushing out the door in the morning, grab an orange and take it with you.

One of the advantages of doing your own baking is that you have more control over the ingredients and can tailor the recipes to provide more nutritional punch. When making muffins or breads, stir in some skim milk powder as a concentrated calcium source. Evaporated milk has double the calcium of ordinary milk, and can be used as a substitute in most recipes.

Another way to get more calcium, especially if you are lactose-intolerant, is to substitute one-quarter soy flour for regular flour in a recipe and add dried figs, dates or apricots to enrich baked treats. Since calcium and iron are available from molasses, use it to sweeten baking wherever possible, instead of sugar or honey.

Granola Bars

Makes 16 squares

Quick and easy to make, these good-for-you bars contain molasses, almonds, dried figs and sesame seeds—all calcium sources. Handy as a portable breakfast, these bars can also be packed in a lunch and served with yogurt or a glass of milk for a great calcium meal.

2 cups	**toasted flakes of corn cereal**	**500 mL**
1 cup	**quick-cooking rolled oats**	**250 mL**
1/2 cup	**toasted chopped almonds**	**125 mL**
1/2 cup	**chopped dried figs**	**125 mL**
1/2 cup	**sesame seeds**	**125 mL**
1/2 tsp	**cinnamon**	**2 mL**
Pinch	**salt**	**Pinch**
1/3 cup	**molasses**	**75 mL**
1	**egg**	**1**

Parchment paper is available in cookware stores and some grocery stores.

1. Preheat oven to 350°F (180°C). Line 8-inch (2 L) square cake pan with parchment paper.
2. In mixing bowl, crush cereal using your hands or base of small bowl until flakes become coarse crumbs. Stir in oats, almonds, figs, sesame seeds, cinnamon and salt.
3. In measuring cup, measure molasses; beat in egg. Stir egg mixture into cereal mixture, combining well, using hands if necessary to mix. Pack firmly into prepared pan.
4. Bake in 350°F (180°C) oven for 20 to 25 minutes or until crisp around edges. Let cool for about 15 minutes. Loosen edges with knife; lift out and, using sharp knife, cut into 16 squares. Squares may be stored in airtight container for up to 2 days. For longer storage, wrap well and freeze for up to 2 months.

Per square	
CALCIUM	41 mg
VITAMIN D	2 IU
Calories	121
Protein	4 g
Fat	5 g
Carbohydrate	16 g
Dietary Fiber	2 g
Sodium	43 mg
Magnesium	43 mg

Triple-Calcium, Freeze-Ahead Bran Muffins

The ultimate in convenience, this calcium-rich batter can be made ahead, spooned into muffin cups and frozen, ready to pop into the oven at a moment's notice. They're yummy, too!

Makes 18 large muffins

2 cups	natural bran	500 mL
1 1/2 cups	all-purpose flour	375 mL
1/2 cup	soy flour or all-purpose flour	125 mL
1/2 cup	granulated sugar	125 mL
1 1/2 tsp	baking soda	7 mL
1 tsp	salt	5 mL
1 tsp	cinnamon	5 mL
2	eggs	2
1	can (385 mL) 2% evaporated milk	1
3/4 cup	molasses	175 mL
2/3 cup	vegetable oil	150 mL
1/2 cup	chopped dates	125 mL
1/2 cup	chopped dried figs	125 mL

Look for soy flour in health food stores and the health food section of some supermarkets.

1. In large bowl, stir together bran, all-purpose flour, soy flour, sugar, baking soda, salt and cinnamon.
2. In separate bowl, whisk together eggs, milk, molasses and oil.
3. Stir egg mixture into bran mixture just until moistened. Stir in dates and figs.
4. Spoon batter into 18 paper-lined large muffin cups, filling each two-thirds full. Cover and freeze until ready to bake. To bake from frozen state, bake in 400°F (200°C) oven for 30 to 35 minutes or until firm to touch. Or bake immediately in 400°F (200°C) oven for 25 to 30 minutes, or until firm to touch.

Per muffin	
CALCIUM	110 mg
VITAMIN D	21 IU
Calories	243
Protein	6 g
Fat	10 g
Carbohydrate	37 g
Dietary Fiber	4 g
Sodium	261 mg
Magnesium	68 mg

Chocolate-Almond Bread Pudding Muffins

Makes 18 muffins

All things old come around again. Bread pudding is no exception. This comfort dessert has acquired new chic, especially in coffee houses, served with steaming cups of Cocoa (p. 37) or Cappuccino (p. 36). You, too, can create the same ambience for your breakfast with a minimum of fuss and expense.

2 1/2 cups	**2% evaporated milk or lactose-reduced milk**	**625 mL**
3	**eggs**	**3**
1 cup	**granulated sugar**	**250 mL**
1/3 cup	**cocoa**	**75 mL**
1 tbsp	**grated orange rind**	**15 mL**
1 tsp	**vanilla extract**	**5 mL**
1/2 tsp	**almond extract**	**2 mL**
8 cups	**cubed white bread**	**2 L**
1/2 cup	**chopped almonds or mixture of almonds and hazelnuts**	**125 mL**

1. Preheat oven to 375°F (190°C). Spray 18 muffin cups with nonstick cooking spray or line with paper muffin-cup liners.
2. In large bowl, gradually whisk milk into eggs. In separate bowl, stir sugar and cocoa together. Whisk a little milk mixture into cocoa mixture to make smooth paste; whisk cocoa mixture into milk mixture. Whisk in orange rind, vanilla extract and almond extract until smooth. Stir in bread and almonds. Let stand for 5 to 10 minutes.
3. Divide mixture evenly among 18 prepared muffin cups. Bake in 375°F (190°C) oven for 30 minutes or until puffed and firm to touch. Let cool on racks for at least 5 minutes before serving. May be served warm or at room temperature. Bread pudding muffins keep for up to 1 day in refrigerator. For longer storage, wrap well and freeze for up to 1 month.

Per muffin	
CALCIUM	124 mg
VITAMIN D	32 IU
Calories	152
Protein	6 g
Fat	4 g
Carbohydrate	23 g
Dietary Fiber	1 g
Sodium	130 mg
Magnesium	24 mg

Couscous with Apricots and Dates

A staple of Moroccan cooking, couscous has gained popularity in this country. For good reason. This North African pasta lends itself to a variety of flavorsome pilafs enhanced with the addition of dried fruits. Although it makes an alternative to porridge at breakfast, this couscous dish is just as good at other mealtimes as an accompaniment to poultry and pork.

Makes 2 cups (500 mL)

1/2 cup	**couscous**	**125 mL**
2 tbsp	**chopped dried apricots**	**25 mL**
2 tbsp	**chopped dates**	**25 mL**
1 tbsp	**chopped almonds**	**15 mL**
1 tbsp	**instant skim milk powder**	**15 mL**
1 tbsp	**orange juice**	**15 mL**
Pinch	**salt**	**Pinch**
1/2 cup	**boiling water**	**125 mL**

To increase the calcium in your diet, stir 1 tbsp (15 mL) of skim milk powder into a recipe.

1. In small bowl, combine couscous, apricots, dates, almonds, milk powder, orange juice and salt. Pour boiling water over couscous mixture; let stand for 4 minutes, covered, or until liquid has been absorbed.
2. Fluff couscous with fork. Serve at once.

Per 1/2 cup (125 mL)	
CALCIUM	29 mg
VITAMIN D	4 IU
Calories	130
Protein	4 g
Fat	1 g
Carbohydrate	26 g
Dietary Fiber	2 g
Sodium	11 mg
Magnesium	18 mg

Whole Grain Fig Bread

Makes one 9- x 5-inch (2 L) loaf, 12 slices

Even the novice baker can produce delicious calcium-rich results with this easy bread. You can toast it and serve it with preserves or cheese for a breakfast or teatime treat. Or try it warm from the oven with soups and salads.

1 cup	**all-purpose flour**	**250 mL**
1 cup	**soy flour or all-purpose flour**	**250 mL**
1 cup	**whole wheat flour**	**250 mL**
1 cup	**quick-cooking rolled oats**	**250 mL**
1 cup	**natural bran**	**250 mL**
3/4 cup	**chopped dried figs**	**175 mL**
1/2 cup	**toasted chopped almonds**	**125 mL**
1/3 cup	**sesame seeds**	**75 mL**
1/4 cup	**instant skim milk powder**	**50 mL**
2 tsp	**baking powder**	**10 mL**
1 tsp	**baking soda**	**5 mL**
1 tsp	**salt**	**5 mL**
1 1/2 cups	**skim milk**	**375 mL**
1/3 cup	**molasses**	**75 mL**
2 tbsp	**sesame seeds**	**25 mL**

1. Preheat oven to 350°F (180°C). Line 9- x 5-inch (2 L) loaf pan with waxed or parchment paper.
2. In bowl, stir together all-purpose flour, soy flour, whole wheat flour, oats, bran, figs, almonds, 1/3 cup (75 mL) sesame seeds, milk powder, baking powder, baking soda and salt.
3. Stir in milk and molasses just until dry ingredients are moistened.

Per slice	
CALCIUM	154 mg
VITAMIN D	19 IU
Calories	266
Protein	12 g
Fat	8 g
Carbohydrate	43 g
Dietary Fiber	7 g
Sodium	363 mg
Magnesium	131 mg

4. Spoon batter into prepared loaf pan. Sprinkle with the 2 tbsp (25 mL) sesame seeds.
5. Bake in 350°F (180°C) oven for 40 to 50 minutes or until tester inserted in center comes out clean. Let cool on rack. Keeps well, covered and refrigerated, for 2 days. For longer storage, wrap well and freeze for up to 3 months.

Fruit and Noodle Casserole

Makes two 10-inch (3 L) bundt pans or two 13- x 9-inch (3.5 L) baking dishes, 24 servings

As you can see from the number of servings, this is a great recipe for a crowd! The casserole can be served warm or at room temperature. It can be made ahead and refrigerated. It tastes heavenly. In fact, it reminds me of a fruited noodle cheesecake with none of the bother. Serve it with ham or sausages, fruit salad and assorted breads for brunch —you'll have a wonderful party!

CASSEROLE:

1	container (500 g) 1% cottage cheese	1
3/4 cup	granulated sugar	175 mL
1 tbsp	grated orange rind	15 mL
5	eggs	5
4 cups	2% evaporated milk or milk	1 L
1 tbsp	cinnamon	15 mL
1 tsp	vanilla extract	5 mL
Pinch	salt	Pinch
3	apples, cored, peeled and thinly sliced	3
1 cup	mixed chopped dried apricots, figs and dates	250 mL
1	pkg (375 g) broad egg noodles	1

TOPPING:

2 cups	fresh brown bread crumbs	500 mL
1/2 cup	chopped almonds	125 mL
1/2 cup	packed brown sugar	125 mL
1/4 cup	melted butter	50 mL
2 tsp	ground cardamom	10 mL

1. Preheat oven to 350°F (180°C). Spray two 10-inch (3 L) bundt pans (or two 13- x 9-inch /3.5 L baking dishes) with nonstick cooking spray.

Per serving	
CALCIUM	166 mg
VITAMIN D	38 IU
Calories	237
Protein	10 g
Fat	6 g
Carbohydrate	36 g
Dietary Fiber	3 g
Sodium	259 mg
Magnesium	34 mg

2. Casserole: In food processor, purée cottage cheese, sugar and rind until smooth. Add eggs, one at a time, combining after adding each one.
3. Transfer cheese mixture to large mixing bowl. Whisk in milk, cinnamon, vanilla and salt. Fold in apples and dried fruit.
4. In large pot of boiling salted water, cook noodles according to package directions. Rinse under cold running water, drain thoroughly and stir into cottage cheese mixture.
5. Divide mixture evenly into two prepared pans.
6. Topping: In bowl, combine bread crumbs, almonds, brown sugar, butter and cardamom until well mixed. Sprinkle mixture evenly over tops of two casseroles.
7. Bake in 350°F (180°C) oven for 1 hour or until set and golden brown around edges. Let cool on racks. Once cool, if using bundt pan, loosen edges with knife and unmold onto serving platter. If using 13- x 9-inch (3.5 L) baking dishes, leave in baking dishes.

Bone-Building Porridge

Makes 2 cups (500 mL), 2 servings

Porridge never tasted so good! By cooking with milk, milk solids, dried fruit and molasses, you have a rich calcium start to the day.

1 1/2 cups	**2% milk**	**375 mL**
2/3 cup	**quick-cooking rolled oats**	**150 mL**
2 tbsp	**dried currants**	**25 mL**
2 tbsp	**instant skim milk powder**	**25 mL**
1 tbsp	**molasses**	**15 mL**
1/2 tsp	**cinnamon**	**2 mL**
Pinch	**salt**	**Pinch**

1. In small saucepan, combine milk, oats, currants, milk powder, molasses, cinnamon and salt. Bring to a boil, stirring. Reduce heat to low; cook for 1 minute, stirring. [Microwave directions: In 8-cup (2 L) microwave-safe container, combine milk, oats, currants, milk powder, molasses, cinnamon and salt. Microwave at High for 4 minutes. Stir; let stand for 1 minute before serving.]

VARIATION:
Substitute 1/4 cup (50 mL) chopped dried figs for the currants; substitute maple syrup for the molasses.

Per serving

CALCIUM	322 mg
VITAMIN D	83 IU
Calories	247
Protein	12 g
Fat	4 g
Carbohydrate	42 g
Dietary Fiber	4 g
Sodium	119 mg
Magnesium	79 mg

Rice Pudding To Go

Here's an old-fashioned favorite with a new look. Served in individual muffin papers, rice pudding can tag along for breakfast or be packed in lunches. Using 2% evaporated milk gives twice the calcium as regular milk and provides a creamy consistency without the fat.

Makes 3 cups (750 mL), 6 servings

1/2 cup	**short-grain (Arborio) rice**	**125 mL**
2 cups	**water**	**500 mL**
1 cup	**2% evaporated milk**	**250 mL**
1 cup	**milk**	**250 mL**
3 tbsp	**granulated sugar**	**50 mL**
2 tsp	**grated lemon rind**	**10 mL**
1	**cinnamon stick**	**1**
1/4 tsp	**salt**	**1 mL**

Look for Arborio rice in the rice section of supermarkets or in Italian markets.

1. In small saucepan, bring rice and water to boil. Reduce heat to medium-low; simmer, covered, for 20 minutes or until tender.
2. Stir in evaporated milk, milk, sugar, lemon rind, cinnamon stick and salt; bring to boil. Reduce heat to medium-low; cook, uncovered, for 30 minutes, stirring frequently.
3. Remove cinnamon stick. Serve pudding immediately. Or spoon pudding into individual containers lined with muffin papers; cover and refrigerate until ready to serve. Rice pudding will keep for 2 days if covered and refrigerated.

Per serving	
CALCIUM	169 mg
VITAMIN D	45 IU
Calories	140
Protein	6 g
Fat	1 g
Carbohydrate	26 g
Dietary Fiber	trace
Sodium	163 mg
Magnesium	20 mg

Baked Salmon Fondue

Makes 6 servings

A simplified version of a soufflé, this fondue can be assembled ahead, ready to pop into the oven. Serve with Calcium Greens (p. 85) dressed with Tarragon Vinaigrette (p. 88) for a calcium-rich brunch or supper.

4	eggs	4
3 cups	milk, lactose-reduced milk or soy beverage	750 mL
2 tbsp	salad dressing	25 mL
2 tsp	Dijon mustard	10 mL
1/2 tsp	black pepper	2 mL
6 cups	coarse bread crumbs	1.5 L
2	cans (each 7 1/2 oz/213 g) salmon	2
2 cups	shredded Swiss cheese	500 mL
1/3 cup	chopped fresh dill	75 mL

To make coarse bread crumbs, cube and measure bread. Then place in food processor or blender to make coarse crumbs.

Swiss cheese is higher in calcium than Cheddar cheese.

1. Grease 8-cup (2 L) baking dish or spray with nonstick cooking spray.
2. In mixing bowl, whisk together eggs, milk, salad dressing, mustard and pepper until well combined. Stir in bread crumbs. Let stand for 10 minutes.
3. Meanwhile, drain salmon; discard skin. Using fork, mash bones and flake salmon; combine with 1 1/2 cups (375 mL) of the cheese and the dill. Set aside.
4. Stir salmon mixture into bread mixture, combining well. Spoon into prepared baking dish. Sprinkle with remaining cheese. (Casserole may be assembled to this point, covered, refrigerated and ready for baking up to 4 hours later.)
5. Bake in 350°F (180°C) oven for 40 to 45 minutes or until puffed, golden brown and firm to touch. Serve immediately.

Per serving	
CALCIUM	629 mg
VITAMIN D	205 IU
Calories	391
Protein	27 g
Fat	20 g
Carbohydrate	24 g
Dietary Fiber	trace
Sodium	523 mg
Magnesium	48 mg

Scones with Cheddar Cheese

A teatime classic, these melt-in-your-mouth scones are sublime served warm with a spreading of cream cheese and a dollop of Cranberry Orange Chutney *(p. 43)* *or Rhubarb, Fig and Ginger Chutney* *(p. 47)**.*

Makes about 12 scones

2 cups	all-purpose flour	500 mL
2 tbsp	instant skim milk powder (optional)	25 mL
2 tsp	cream of tartar	10 mL
1/2 tsp	baking soda	2 mL
1/2 tsp	salt	2 mL
1/3 cup	shortening	75 mL
1/2 cup	shredded old Cheddar cheese	125 mL
1/2 cup	milk or lactose-reduced milk	125 mL
1/2 cup	plain yogurt	125 mL

1. Preheat oven to 425°F (220°C). Line baking sheet with parchment paper.
2. In mixing bowl, stir together flour, skim milk powder (if using), cream of tartar, baking soda and salt.
3. Using pastry cutter or two knives, cut shortening into flour mixture until mixture resembles coarse crumbs. Stir in cheese.
4. Using fork, stir in milk and yogurt just until moistened. Using lightly floured hands, knead dough to form ball.
5. Turn dough out onto sheet of waxed paper; pat into circle about 1 1/2-inch (4 cm) thick. Using 1 1/2-inch (4 cm) round cookie cutter, cut out about 12 scones. Reroll dough if necessary and cut again.
6. Arrange scones on prepared baking sheet. Bake in 425°F (220°C) oven for 10 to 12 minutes or until browned. Serve warm. Scones are best served immediately, but may be baked a day ahead and rewarmed. For longer storage, wrap well and freeze for up to 3 months.

For an extra calcium boost, dip scones into a bowl of sesame seeds before baking.

Dip cookie cutter into a bowl of vegetable oil each time you cut out dough for easy release of the scone.

Per scone	
CALCIUM	77 mg
VITAMIN D	7 IU
Calories	157
Protein	4 g
Fat	7 g
Carbohydrate	18 g
Dietary Fiber	1 g
Sodium	190 mg
Magnesium	10 mg

Orange Scones with Almonds and Dates

Makes about 16 scones

Scones are always popular whether for breakfast, a snack or served with cheese for lunch. These ones have an extra boost of calcium with skim milk powder, soy flour, yogurt, dates and almonds. Serve scones with your favorite spread.

1 1/2 cups	all-purpose flour	375 mL
1/2 cup	soy flour or all-purpose flour	125 mL
2 tbsp	granulated sugar	25 mL
2 tbsp	instant skim milk powder (optional)	25 mL
2 tsp	cream of tartar	10 mL
2 tsp	grated orange rind	10 mL
1/2 tsp	salt	2 mL
1/2 tsp	baking soda	2 mL
1/2 cup	chopped dates	125 mL
1/3 cup	shortening	75 mL
1/2 cup	plain yogurt	125 mL
1/2 cup	orange juice	125 mL
1/4 cup	chopped almonds	50 mL

1. Preheat oven to 425°F (220°C). Line baking sheet with parchment paper.
2. In mixing bowl, stir together all-purpose flour, soy flour, sugar, skim milk powder, cream of tartar, orange rind, salt and baking soda. Stir in dates.
3. Using pastry cutter or two knives, cut shortening into flour mixture until mixture resembles coarse crumbs.

Per scone

CALCIUM	36 mg
VITAMIN D	2 IU
Calories	132
Protein	4 g
Fat	6 g
Carbohydrate	18 g
Dietary Fiber	1 g
Sodium	118 mg
Magnesium	22 mg

4. Stir in yogurt and juice just until moistened.
5. On sheet of waxed paper, pat dough to 1 1/2-inch (4 cm) thickness. Using 1 1/2-inch (4 cm) round cookie cutter, cut out about 16 scones. Dip each scone into bowl of almonds, gently pressing top surface of scone into nuts.
6. Bake in 425°F (220°C) oven for 10 to 12 minutes or until browned. Scones are best served fresh from the oven, but they may be baked a day ahead and rewarmed. For longer storage, wrap well and freeze for up to 3 months.

Tex-Mex Fondue

Makes 4 servings

You will often see versions of this recipe in old cookbooks; these fondues were considered a good way to use up stale bread and bits of old cheese. Although humble in origin, this is a comforting casserole with all the benefits of make-ahead ease that's ideal for breakfast, brunch or lunch. You can serve this warm with salsa.

4	**eggs**	**4**
3 cups	**skim milk**	**750 mL**
2 cups	**shredded old Cheddar cheese (about 4 oz/113 g)**	**500 mL**
1/4 cup	**instant skim milk powder**	**50 mL**
1/4 cup	**salsa**	**50 mL**
2 tsp	**Dijon mustard**	**10 mL**
Pinch	**nutmeg**	**Pinch**
6 cups	**coarse bread crumbs (preferably day-old brown)**	**1.5 L**

1. Grease 8-cup (2 L) baking dish or spray with nonstick cooking spray.
2. Whisk together eggs, milk, cheese, skim milk powder, salsa, mustard and nutmeg. Fold in bread crumbs, stirring to combine well.
3. Spoon egg mixture into prepared baking dish; cover and refrigerate for at least 30 minutes or overnight to allow bread to soak up liquid.
4. Bake in 350°F (180°C) oven for 40 to 45 minutes or until puffed and golden brown. Serve immediately.

Per serving	
CALCIUM	550 mg
VITAMIN D	117 IU
Calories	397
Protein	25 g
Fat	18 g
Carbohydrate	35 g
Dietary Fiber	5 g
Sodium	718 mg
Magnesium	43 mg

Calcium Granola

Sprinkled on cereal or nibbled as a snack, this is a yummy granola enriched with the goodness of calcium from almonds, sesame seeds, molasses and figs. Lower in fat than some commercial brands, this granola makes a great start to the day.

Makes about 10 cups (2.5 L)

7 cups	quick-cooking rolled oats	1.75 L
1 cup	natural bran	250 mL
1 cup	sweetened coconut flakes	250 mL
1 cup	unblanched almonds or hazelnuts	250 mL
1/2 cup	sesame seeds	125 mL
1/2 cup	shelled roasted salted sunflower seeds	125 mL
3/4 cup	molasses	175 mL
1/2 cup	water	125 mL
1/2 cup	vegetable oil	125 mL
1 tsp	vanilla extract	5 mL
1 tsp	salt	5 mL
1 cup	chopped dried fruit (figs, dates, apricots or mixture)	250 mL

Of all dried fruits, dried figs contain the most calcium.

1. Preheat oven to 350°F (180°C). Grease 17 1/2- x 11 1/2-inch (3 L) jelly roll pan or line with parchment paper.
2. In large mixing bowl, stir together oats, bran, coconut, almonds, sesame seeds and sunflower seeds.
3. In small bowl, whisk together molasses, water, oil, vanilla and salt.
4. Pour molasses mixture over oat mixture, stirring to combine. Spoon onto jelly roll pan, smoothing out. Bake in 350°F (180°C) oven for about 30 minutes or until deep golden brown and fragrant.
5. Let cool; stir in figs. Store refrigerated in glass jars for up to 1 week. Freeze for up to 3 months.

Per 1/2 cup (125 mL)

CALCIUM	77 mg
Calories	317
Protein	8 g
Fat	16 g
Carbohydrate	39 g
Dietary Fiber	6 g
Sodium	156 mg
Magnesium	111 mg

Whole Wheat Calcium-Yeast Bread

Makes two 9- x 5-inch (2 L) loaves, 24 slices

Once you have tried this full-flavored bread, you will never settle for commercial bread again. This is great toasted for breakfast or served with hearty soups.

3 cups	lukewarm water	750 mL
2	pkgs (each 8 g) traditional active dry yeast	2
2 tsp	granulated sugar	10 mL
1 cup	natural bran	250 mL
1 cup	soy flour	250 mL
3/4 cup	instant skim milk powder	175 mL
1/2 cup	sesame seeds	125 mL
1/3 cup	molasses	75 mL
1/4 cup	vegetable oil	50 mL
1 tbsp	salt	15 mL
3 cups	(approx) all-purpose flour	750 mL
3 cups	(approx) whole wheat flour	750 mL

One package of yeast is about 1 tablespoon (15 mL).

1. Grease or spray with nonstick cooking spray two 9- x 5-inch (2 L) loaf pans.
2. Rinse large mixing bowl in warm water. Pour in the lukewarm water; sprinkle with yeast and sugar. Let stand in warm place for 10 minutes.
3. Whisk in bran, soy flour, skim milk powder, sesame seeds, molasses, oil and salt until combined.
4. Gradually whisk in all-purpose flour and whole wheat flour until dough starts to stiffen, stirring in enough flour to make a stiff dough. Knead in enough flour to make a smooth, elastic dough that's springy to the touch, about 5 minutes.

Per slice	
CALCIUM	57 mg
VITAMIN D	9 IU
Calories	186
Protein	8 g
Fat	5 g
Carbohydrate	31 g
Dietary Fiber	4 g
Sodium	305 mg
Magnesium	68 mg

5. Form dough into ball; turn dough into oiled bowl. Cover with plastic wrap. For fast rising, place bowl in larger bowl of warm water.
6. When dough has doubled in size, about 40 minutes, punch down. Divide dough into 2 equal portions; pat into two prepared loaf pans. Set in warm spot; let rise until double in size, about 40 minutes.
7. Meanwhile, preheat oven to 375°F (190°C). Bake risen loaves for 35 to 45 minutes or until deep golden brown and firm to touch. Let cool on racks for 15 minutes before removing from pans. Loaves keep well at room temperature for up to 2 days. For longer storage, wrap well and freeze for up to 3 months.

Orange, Sesame and Almond Loaf

Makes one 9- x 5-inch (2 L) loaf, 12 slices

A cross between a pound cake and a coffee cake, this is a luscious sweet bread to serve for a brunch or snack. Soy flour, orange juice, yogurt, sesame seeds and almonds all contribute calcium.

1 cup	granulated sugar	250 mL
1/2 cup	butter	125 mL
1 tbsp	grated orange rind	15 mL
2	eggs	2
1/2 cup	1% plain yogurt	125 mL
1/2 cup	orange juice	125 mL
1 1/2 cups	all-purpose flour	375 mL
1/2 cup	soy flour or all-purpose flour	125 mL
1/4 cup	sesame seeds	50 mL
1/4 cup	sliced almonds	50 mL
1 tsp	baking powder	5 mL
1 tsp	baking soda	5 mL
1/2 tsp	salt	2 mL

GLAZE:

1/3 cup	granulated sugar	75 mL
1/4 cup	orange juice	50 mL
2 tbsp	sliced almonds	25 mL

For those people who are lactose-intolerant, substitute shortening for butter. Yogurt may be tolerated; if not, use an equivalent amount of orange juice instead.

1. Preheat oven to 350°F (180°C). Line 9- x 5-inch (2 L) loaf pan with waxed paper.
2. In mixing bowl, using electric mixer, beat sugar, butter and orange rind together until fluffy. Beat in eggs, one at a time, then yogurt and orange juice. Set aside.

Per slice	
CALCIUM	58 mg
VITAMIN D	6 IU
Calories	284
Protein	7 g
Fat	12 g
Carbohydrate	39 g
Dietary Fiber	1 g
Sodium	314 mg
Magnesium	39 mg

3. In separate bowl, stir together all-purpose flour, soy flour, sesame seeds, almonds, baking powder, baking soda and salt.
4. Using electric mixer, gradually beat flour mixture into creamed mixture. Spoon batter into prepared loaf pan. Bake in 350°F (180°C) oven for 50 to 60 minutes or until golden brown and toothpick inserted in center comes out clean.
5. Glaze: In measuring cup, whisk together sugar and orange juice. Pour over loaf while loaf is still warm. Sprinkle evenly with almonds.

Chapter 2

Beverages

Coffee has become the beverage of the 1990s—with cappuccino, latte, café au lait and espresso heading the list in coffee bars and restaurants, with old-fashioned regular bringing up the rear. Although the Osteoporosis Society recommends moderate caffeine consumption (no more than 3 cups of coffee, tea or cola beverages per day) milky coffees like cappuccino, café au lait and latte are preferable. They use a substantial amount of milk as an ingredient, thus boosting calcium intake. When made with decaffeinated coffee, these drinks do not have the diuretic effect of regular caffeinated coffee which causes a small calcium loss from the body.

Of course, there are many adults and children who don't drink coffee and would prefer a steaming cup of cocoa or a frothy milk shake jam-packed with the goodness of seasonal fruit. These beverages can be satisfying and delicious, and a great way to get calcium. By using evaporated milk, you also acquire the richness of cream without the fat and you double the calcium! That's a bonus. Low-fat milk shakes, including soy shakes, acquire their lush decadent taste and texture not from high-fat ice cream or cream, but from the addition of puréed fruit while maintaining low fat by using skim milk, 1% milk or low-fat soft tofu.

Cappuccino

Makes 1 serving

By using evaporated milk, you get twice as much calcium as regular milk.

Per serving	
CALCIUM	353 mg
VITAMIN D	93 IU
Calories	120
Protein	10 g
Fat	3 g
Carbohydrate	15 g
Dietary Fiber	0 g
Sodium	143 mg
Magnesium	37 mg

You don't need a fancy coffee machine to make this popular beverage.

1/2 cup	2% evaporated milk	125 mL
1	packet (1.5 g) instant espresso granules	1
1/4 cup	boiling water	50 mL
Pinch	cinnamon	Pinch
	Granulated sugar	

1. In small saucepan, heat milk over medium-high heat, whisking, until hot and frothy.
2. In serving mug, dissolve espresso granules in boiling water. Stir in hot milk. Sprinkle with cinnamon. Add sugar to taste.

Mocaccino

Makes 1 serving

Per serving	
CALCIUM	709 mg
VITAMIN D	187 IU
Calories	297
Protein	20 g
Fat	6 g
Carbohydrate	43 g
Dietary Fiber	1 g
Sodium	311 mg
Magnesium	71 mg

A cross between cocoa and coffee, this is a great treat for a leisurely breakfast or a pick-me-up later in the day.

1 tbsp	granulated sugar	15 mL
2 tsp	unsweetened cocoa powder	10 mL
1 tsp	instant coffee granules	5 mL
1	cinnamon stick	1
1 cup	2% evaporated milk	250 mL

1. In saucepan, whisk together sugar, cocoa and coffee until well blended. Add cinnamon stick.
2. Over medium-high heat, gradually whisk in milk until well combined. Cook for 3 to 4 minutes or until mocaccino is hot. Remove cinnamon stick. Serve beverage hot.

Cocoa

Nothing tastes better on a chilly day than a steaming cup of cocoa. When time is tight, cocoa provides a mini-meal-in-a-hurry.

Makes 1 serving

1 tbsp	**unsweetened cocoa powder**	**15 mL**
1 tbsp	**granulated sugar**	**15 mL**
1 cup	**milk (skim or milk of your choice)**	**250 mL**

1. In saucepan, combine cocoa powder and sugar. Pour 2 tbsp (25 mL) of the milk into cocoa mixture; whisk until smooth. Gradually pour in remaining milk, whisking until well combined.
2. Cook cocoa over medium-high heat, whisking frequently until hot, about 3 minutes. [Microwave directions: Microwave cocoa in microwave-safe cup at High for 2 minutes. Whisk and serve.]

Per serving	
CALCIUM	308 mg
VITAMIN D	85 IU
Calories	167
Protein	9 g
Fat	4 g
Carbohydrate	27 g
Dietary Fiber	2 g
Sodium	164 mg
Magnesium	34 mg

Strawberry Milk Shake

Makes about 2 cups (500 mL), 2 servings

Per serving	
CALCIUM	161 mg
VITAMIN D	50 IU
Calories	97
Protein	4 g
Fat	2 g
Carbohydrate	17 g
Dietary Fiber	2 g
Sodium	62 mg
Magnesium	25 mg

Milk shakes are the one way I can get my seven-year-old daughter, Alexa, to drink milk. She hates milk in all other colors and flavors. It helps that I include in the shakes the frozen strawberries that she helped me pick in the summer. To produce a smooth, creamy treat, a blender works better than a food processor. However, a food processor can be used, too.

1 cup	**strawberries (fresh or frozen)**	**250 mL**
1 cup	**skim milk**	**250 mL**
1 tbsp	**(approx) granulated sugar**	**15 mL**
1/2 tsp	**vanilla extract (optional)**	**2 mL**

1. In blender, add strawberries, milk, sugar to taste and vanilla (if using). Blend until smooth.

Strawberry-Banana Milk Shake

Makes about 2 cups (500 mL), 2 servings

Per serving	
CALCIUM	157 mg
VITAMIN D	50 IU
Calories	97
Protein	5 g
Fat	2 g
Carbohydrate	17 g
Dietary Fiber	1 g
Sodium	62 mg
Magnesium	29 mg

Here's a thicker, creamy version of the Strawberry Milk Shake (above).

1 cup	**skim milk**	**250 mL**
1/2 cup	**strawberries (fresh or frozen)**	**125 mL**
Half	**banana**	**Half**
1 tsp	**(approx) granulated sugar**	**5 mL**

1. In blender, add milk, strawberries, banana and sugar to taste. Blend until smooth.

Strawberry Tofu Shake

Makes about 3 cups (750 mL), 2 servings

Although milk shakes can be made with soy beverage, shakes made with tofu may be a better source of calcium than those with soy beverage. Tofu containing calcium sulfate or calcium chloride will contain more calcium than the products prepared without these coagulating ingredients. Check the ingredient list on the package to determine the type of coagulant used.

1 cup	**drained silken soft tofu**	**250 mL**
1 cup	**orange juice**	**250 mL**
1/2 cup	**strawberries (fresh or frozen)**	**125 mL**
Half	**banana**	**Half**

1. In blender, add tofu, orange juice, strawberries and banana. Blend until smooth.

Per serving	
CALCIUM	87 mg
Calories	160
Protein	8 g
Fat	3 g
Carbohydrate	25 g
Dietary Fiber	2 g
Sodium	19 mg
Magnesium	24 mg

Chapter 3

Sauces and Condiments

Sauces and condiments easily lend themselves to being enriched by ingredients containing calcium. For instance, cheese sauce provides a double dose of calcium with cheese and milk. When combined with broccoli, the broccoli and cheese sauce delivers a great calcium package.

Yogurt is an ideal low-fat base for sauces and dressings—both sweet and savory. What's more, in many cases, yogurt can be digested by lactose-intolerant people who are unable to consume milk products in other forms. Use it as a sweet sauce to complement fruit and pudding desserts. With added herbs, yogurt makes an easy sauce for main-course items.

Chutneys by definition are a sweet-and-sour combination of fruits and/or vegetables cooked with spices and vinegar to a jam-like consistency. Why not include the calcium choices of dried figs, dried apricots, dates or raisins with the crunch of almonds? There are numerous other preserves where these dried fruits and nuts are included. Experiment with preserves and sauces to create a diet that incorporates more calcium.

Cheese Sauce Mix

Makes about 1 cup (250 mL)

Per 1/3 cup (75 mL)	
CALCIUM	480 mg
VITAMIN D	50 IU
Calories	251
Protein	16 g
Fat	16 g
Carbohydrate	11 g
Dietary Fiber	0 g
Sodium	355 mg
Magnesium	27 mg

A useful mix to transform into quick sauces for vegetables or pasta with the triple-calcium combo of cheese, skim milk powder and milk.

1 1/4 cups	**grated old Cheddar cheese**	**300 mL**
1/2 cup	**instant skim milk powder**	**125 mL**
2 tbsp	**cornstarch**	**25 mL**

1. Combine cheese, milk powder and cornstarch in food processor until well mixed. Can be stored in a jar in the refrigerator for up to 1 month.

Cheese Sauce

Makes about 3/4 cup (175 mL)

Per 1/4 cup (50 mL)	
CALCIUM	235 mg
VITAMIN D	38 IU
Calories	109
Protein	7 g
Fat	6 g
Carbohydrate	7 g
Dietary Fiber	0 g
Sodium	149 mg
Magnesium	17 mg

1/3 cup	**Cheese Sauce Mix (above)**	**75 mL**
3/4 cup	**milk**	**175 mL**
Pinch	**each cayenne pepper, nutmeg and salt**	**Pinch**

1. In saucepan, over medium-high heat, whisk Cheese Sauce Mix with milk, cayenne pepper, nutmeg and salt until smooth and thickened, about 1 minute. Serve at once.

Cranberry-Orange Chutney

A jar of this brilliant chutney has many uses. For a dramatic presentation, serve this as the topping for the Savory Cheddar and Orange Cheesecake (p. 51) or spread some cream cheese onto Scones with Cheddar Cheese (p. 25) and top with a little chutney. Of course, this chutney is the perfect accompaniment to roast turkey, too!

Makes about 3 cups (750 mL)

2 cups	cranberries (fresh or frozen)	500 mL
1 cup	packed brown sugar	250 mL
1	onion, chopped	1
3/4 cup	cider vinegar	175 mL
1/2 cup	orange juice	125 mL
1 tbsp	grated orange rind	15 mL
1 tsp	salt	5 mL
1/2 tsp	dry mustard	2 mL
1/2 tsp	ground ginger	2 mL
1/2 tsp	cinnamon	2 mL
1/2 cup	chopped dates	125 mL
1/2 cup	chopped dried figs	125 mL
1/2 cup	toasted chopped almonds	125 mL

You need a stainless-steel saucepan so that acid from the cranberries and vinegar does not react with the metal. Glass saucepans work well, too.

1. In stainless-steel saucepan, combine cranberries, brown sugar, onion, vinegar, orange juice, grated rind, salt, mustard, ginger and cinnamon. Bring to boil; reduce heat to low and simmer chutney, uncovered, for 15 minutes, stirring frequently.
2. Stir in dates, figs and almonds. Continue to cook, uncovered, until chutney has thickened, 5 to 10 minutes.
3. Spoon hot chutney into hot sterilized jars, leaving 1/4-inch (5 mm) headspace; seal; process in boiling water bath for 10 minutes. Alternatively, spoon chutney into sterilized jars and refrigerate for up to 2 weeks; or freeze chutney in plastic containers for up to 6 months. Remember to label and date containers.

Per 2 tbsp (25 mL)	
CALCIUM	26 mg
Calories	80
Protein	1 g
Fat	2 g
Carbohydrate	17 g
Dietary Fiber	1 g
Sodium	100 mg
Magnesium	17 mg

Cucumber-Dill Sauce

Makes about 3 cups (750 mL)

Here is the ideal calcium companion for fish and other seafood. Refreshing, tangy and easy to make, try this sauce as a topping for grilled fish, use it in pitas or serve it as a condiment with vegetarian dishes.

1	**English cucumber**	**1**
2 cups	**1% plain yogurt**	**500 mL**
2 tbsp	**chopped fresh dill**	**25 mL**
1 tbsp	**lemon juice**	**15 mL**
1	**green onion, chopped**	**1**
1/2 tsp	**salt**	**2 mL**
	Pepper	

1. Using coarse side of grater, grate cucumber. Drain in colander for 15 minutes, pressing out any excess moisture.
2. In bowl, stir together cucumber, yogurt, dill, lemon juice, green onion, salt and pepper to taste. Spoon into serving bowl.
3. Cover and refrigerate until serving time. Sauce may be made 1 day ahead; it keeps for 2 days in refrigerator. Stir before serving if separated.

VARIATION:
Stir 2 cloves of garlic (minced) into this sauce to make tzatziki; serve with sliced baguette.

Per 2 tbsp (25 mL)	
CALCIUM	39 mg
Calories	14
Protein	1 g
Fat	trace
Carbohydrate	2 g
Dietary Fiber	trace
Sodium	63 mg
Magnesium	5 mg

Drained Yogurt

Drained yogurt, also called yogurt cheese, will condense to half its original volume within four hours. You can use it plain, as dollops on top of soups and stews. Or you can sweeten and flavor it in different ways for use as sauces to accompany fruit salads, puddings, cakes and pies. It can even be used to make Frozen Lemon Yogurt (p. 156).

Makes 1 1/2 cups (375 mL)

3 cups	**1% plain yogurt**	**750 mL**

1. Line a strainer with cheesecloth, paper towels or coffee filters; place over a bowl.
2. Pour yogurt into lined strainer.
3. Cover with plastic wrap; let drain for at least 2 hours or overnight in refrigerator.

Per 1/4 cup (50 mL)	
CALCIUM	120 mg
Calories	55
Protein	6 g
Fat	1 g
Carbohydrate	6 g
Dietary Fiber	0 g
Sodium	32 mg
Magnesium	10 mg

All-Purpose Yogurt Dessert Sauce

There are a variety of sauces throughout the book using drained yogurt, but this basic sauce can be served with just about any dessert.

Makes 1 cup (250 mL)

1 cup	**Drained Yogurt (yogurt cheese)** (above)	**250 mL**
2 tbsp	**packed brown sugar**	**25 mL**
2 tsp	**vanilla extract, dark rum or imported orange liqueur**	**10 mL**

1. In mixing bowl, whisk together yogurt cheese, brown sugar and vanilla until smooth. Spoon into serving bowl; cover and refrigerate for up to 1 day before serving.

Per 2 tbsp (25 mL)	
CALCIUM	63 mg
Calories	44
Protein	3 g
Fat	1 g
Carbohydrate	6 g
Dietary Fiber	0 g
Sodium	17 mg
Magnesium	6 mg

Marzipan

Makes about 1 cup (250 mL)

Once you have tasted your own homemade marzipan, you will never buy the commercial variety again. For best flavor and freshness, buy unblanched almonds and blanch them yourself. However, if time is tight, use packaged ground almonds.

1 cup	**ground almonds***	**250 mL**
1 cup	**icing sugar**	**250 mL**
2 tbsp	**egg white (about 1 egg white)**	**25 mL**
1 tsp	**almond extract**	**5 mL**
1 tsp	**corn syrup or honey**	**5 mL**

***To blanch almonds, cover 1 1/2 cups unblanched almonds with boiling water. Let stand for 5 minutes. Squeezing almond between thumb and forefinger, almond should pop out of skin. Then grind almonds to make 1 cup (250 mL).**

1. In food processor, combine almonds and icing sugar until well mixed.
2. With motor running, pour egg white, almond extract and corn syrup through feed tube. Process until mixture holds together in a ball. Remove mixture; keep covered in plastic container in refrigerator until ready to use for frosting a cake or for shaping into truffles.

VARIATION:
To use as a frosting, sprinkle marzipan with icing sugar; roll out marzipan between two layers of waxed paper large enough to cover top of cake. Trim any excess. One cup of marzipan is enough to cover top of 9-inch (23 cm) or 10-inch (25 cm) cake.

Per tbsp (15 mL)	
CALCIUM	13 mg
Calories	60
Protein	1 g
Fat	3 g
Carbohydrate	8 g
Dietary Fiber	trace
Sodium	4 mg
Magnesium	15 mg

Rhubarb, Fig and Ginger Chutney

A batch of this irresistible chutney has many uses. It is delicious spread on top of cream cheese and crackers or served as a condiment for any poultry dish. For a spectacular treat, use this chutney as the topping for Savory Cheddar and Orange Cheesecake (p. 51). Rhubarb contains calcium but the calcium is not available to our bodies; therefore, rhubarb cannot be considered a calcium source.

Makes about 4 cups (1 L)

5 cups	chopped rhubarb (fresh or frozen)	1.25 L
1	large onion, chopped	1
1 cup	cider vinegar	250 mL
3/4 cup	brown sugar	175 mL
3/4 cup	granulated sugar	175 mL
1 cup	chopped dried figs	250 mL
1/2 cup	chopped crystallized ginger	125 mL
1/2 tsp	salt	2 mL
1/2 tsp	cinnamon	2 mL
1/2 tsp	ground cloves	2 mL

You need a stainless-steel saucepan so that acid from the rhubarb and vinegar does not react with the metal. Glass saucepans work well, too.

1. In large stainless-steel saucepan over medium-high heat, combine rhubarb, onion, vinegar, brown sugar, granulated sugar, figs, ginger, salt, cinnamon and cloves.
2. Bring to boil; reduce heat to low and simmer, uncovered, stirring frequently until thickened, about 30 to 35 minutes.
3. Ladle chutney into hot sterilized jars, leaving 1/4-inch (5 mm) headspace; seal. Process in boiling water bath for 10 minutes. Alternatively, jars of chutney may be stored in refrigerator (without processing in boiling water bath) for up to 2 weeks; or chutney may be frozen in plastic containers for up to 6 months.

Per 2 tbsp (25 mL)	
CALCIUM	21 mg
Calories	69
Protein	trace
Fat	trace
Carbohydrate	18 g
Dietary Fiber	1 g
Sodium	41 mg
Magnesium	9 mg

Ricotta-Apricot Filling or Frosting

Makes 2 1/2 cups (625 mL)

This is a not-too-sweet filling or frosting bursting with flavor and calcium. If you are using it to frost a cake, leave the apricots out and use them as a garnish on top of the cake. Spread this filling on crêpes, pancakes, jelly rolls or sliced tea breads. It also makes a nice alternative to butter on muffins.

1	**container (500 g) extra-fine ricotta cheese**	**1**
1/2 cup	**chopped dried apricots**	**125 mL**
1/4 cup	**icing sugar**	**50 mL**
2 tbsp	**imported orange liqueur or orange juice**	**25 mL**

1. In mixing bowl, beat together ricotta cheese, apricots, icing sugar and orange liqueur until well blended. Use immediately; or store, covered, in refrigerator for up to 2 days.

Per 2 tbsp (25 mL)	
CALCIUM	51 mg
Calories	58
Protein	3 g
Fat	3 g
Carbohydrate	5 g
Dietary Fiber	trace
Sodium	20 mg
Magnesium	4 mg

Chapter 4

Appetizers

Whenever I think of appetizers, I think of rich spreads and dips, cheese concoctions and fat. But there are other calcium nibbles that don't skimp on taste and are not loaded with fat. The addition of crunchy almonds, hazelnuts and sesame seeds provides a calcium boost to the tempting recipes in this chapter.

Beans, especially soybeans, are a good bet, too, for use in spreads such as hummus. For a quick nibble, canned beans are convenient to have on hand. Other ingredients, such as sardines and salmon (including their bones) lend themselves to a host of sophisticated spreads that are bursting with flavor and calcium. In addition to the great taste and the added benefit of calcium, you'll probably appreciate the fact that these easy appetizers won't break the calorie bank.

Navy Bean Hummus

Makes about 2 cups (500 mL)

Hummus is a spread of Middle Eastern origin, traditionally made with chick-peas. This version has more calcium when made with navy beans or soybeans. Canned soybeans and canned navy beans are available in some supermarkets and health food stores. If using canned beans, do not add salt to the recipe. Serve hummus with crackers, breads or Tortilla Crisps *(p. 53)**.*

2 cups	cooked navy (pea) beans [or 1 can (19 oz/540 mL) soybeans, drained and rinsed]	500 mL
1/4 cup	chopped fresh parsley	50 mL
1/4 cup	lemon juice	50 mL
2 tbsp	olive oil	25 mL
1 tbsp	minced green onion	15 mL
1	clove garlic, minced	1
3/4 tsp	salt	4 mL
1/4 tsp	pepper	1 mL
2 pinches	cayenne pepper	2 pinches

1. In food processor, purée beans, parsley, lemon juice, olive oil, green onion, garlic, salt, pepper and cayenne.

Per 2 tbsp (25 mL)	
CALCIUM	19 mg
Calories	49
Protein	2 g
Fat	2 g
Carbohydrate	6 g
Dietary Fiber	2 g
Sodium	163 mg
Magnesium	14 mg

Savory Cheddar and Orange Cheesecake

This versatile no-bake savory cheesecake makes a dramatic first impression as an orange cheesecake when spread with Cranberry-Orange Chutney (p. 43) or Rhubarb, Fig and Ginger Chutney (p. 47). Impressive in appearance and taste, any leftover cheese mixture can be shaped into cheese truffles and rolled in chopped, toasted almonds or hazelnuts or simply packed into a crock to be served with whole-wheat cocktail biscuits. Serve the cheesecake with assorted crackers and breads.

Makes about 5 cups (1.25 L), serves a crowd

1 lb	**extra old Cheddar cheese, shredded (about 8 cups/2 L shredded)**	**500 g**
8 oz	**light cream cheese**	**250 g**
1/2 cup	**butter, softened**	**125 mL**
1/4 cup	**dry sherry**	**50 mL**
1 tbsp	**grated orange rind**	**15 mL**
2 tsp	**Dijon mustard**	**10 mL**
1/4 tsp	**ground nutmeg**	**1 mL**

TOPPING:

3-4 cups	**chutney**	**750 mL-1 L**

1. Line 8-inch (2 L) springform pan or straight-sided cake pan with plastic wrap.
2. In food processor or in large bowl using electric mixer, beat together Cheddar cheese, cream cheese, butter, sherry, orange rind, mustard and nutmeg until smooth.
3. Spoon cheese mixture into prepared pan. Level top.
4. Cover with plastic wrap and refrigerate for at least 2 hours before serving or for up to 2 days.
5. Topping: To serve, unwrap and invert pan onto serving plate. Remove pan and plastic wrap. Spoon chutney on top.

Per 2 tbsp (25 mL)	
CALCIUM	99 mg
Calories	104
Protein	3 g
Fat	8 g
Carbohydrate	6 g
Dietary Fiber	trace
Sodium	137 mg
Magnesium	6 mg

Cheese Shortbread

Makes about 30

Keep a batch of this shortbread dough in the freezer, ready to slice and bake. These shortbreads are the perfect nibble with a glass of wine.

1 cup	**all-purpose flour**	**250 mL**
1 cup	**shredded old Cheddar cheese (about 2 oz/50 g)**	**250 mL**
1/2 cup	**cold butter, cubed**	**125 mL**
Pinch	**cayenne pepper**	**Pinch**
1 tbsp	**sesame seeds**	**15 mL**

Rolling dough out on waxed paper makes the clean-up easier.

Dough may be sliced and baked from the frozen state at 350°F (180°C) until golden brown.

1. Preheat oven to 350°F (180°C). Line baking sheet with parchment paper.
2. In bowl of food processor, combine flour, cheese, butter and cayenne. Process for 30 seconds or until well blended and mixture starts forming a ball.
3. Form dough into log that's 1 1/2 inches (4 cm) in diameter. Sprinkle with sesame seeds; roll to press sesame seeds to outside.
4. Using sharp knife, slice log at 1/4-inch (5 mm) intervals; arrange on prepared baking sheet. Bake in 350°F (180°C) oven for 20 to 25 minutes or until golden brown. Store in cookie tin for up to 2 days. For longer storage, wrap well and freeze for up to 2 months.

Per piece	
CALCIUM	29 mg
Calories	59
Protein	1 g
Fat	5 g
Carbohydrate	3 g
Dietary Fiber	trace
Sodium	55 mg
Magnesium	3 mg

Tortilla Crisps

A few tortillas can be transformed into fragrant flatbread. They are delectable served on their own, warm from the oven, or used as dippers for Navy Bean Hummus (p. 50).

Makes 32 pieces

4	**10-inch (25 cm) flour tortillas (burrito-size)**	**4**
1	**egg white**	**1**
2 tbsp	**sesame seeds**	**25 mL**

1. Preheat oven to 350°F (180°C). Line baking sheet with parchment paper.
2. Place tortillas on cutting board. Brush egg white over tortillas. Sprinkle each with sesame seeds.
3. Cut each tortilla into eight wedges. Place on prepared baking sheet.
4. Bake in 350°F (180°C) oven for 15 to 20 minutes or until golden.

VARIATION:
To make Parmesan-Rosemary Flatbread, substitute 2 tbsp (25 mL) freshly grated Parmesan cheese and 4 tsp (20 mL) dried rosemary for the sesame seeds.

Per piece	
CALCIUM	12 mg
Calories	28
Protein	1 g
Fat	1 g
Carbohydrate	4 g
Dietary Fiber	trace
Sodium	29 mg
Magnesium	5 mg

Pesto Croustades

Makes about 36 pieces

Always popular whether served as mini-pizzas to a young crowd or as hot appetizers to an older group, these croustades can be assembled and baked immediately or covered and frozen, ready to pop into the oven at a moment's notice.

ALMOND PESTO:

2 cups	fresh parsley leaves	500 mL
1/2 cup	freshly grated Parmesan cheese	125 mL
1/4 cup	toasted slivered almonds	50 mL
2 tbsp	dried basil	25 mL
3	cloves garlic, minced	3
1/2 tsp	salt	2 mL
1/4 tsp	pepper	1 mL
3/4 cup	olive oil	175 mL

CROUSTADES:

1	baguette	1
3/4 cup	oil-packed sun-dried tomatoes	175 mL
2 cups	shredded mozzarella cheese	500 mL

1. Almond Pesto: In food processor, combine parsley, Parmesan cheese, almonds, basil, garlic, salt and pepper; process until finely chopped.
2. With motor running, pour oil through feed tube; process until smooth. Spoon pesto into jar. Refrigerate for up to 1 day; or for longer storage, freeze for up to 2 months.
3. Croustades: Line baking sheet with parchment paper. Slice baguette into 3/4-inch (2 cm) pieces.

Per piece	
CALCIUM	70 mg
Calories	102
Protein	3 g
Fat	8 g
Carbohydrate	6 g
Dietary Fiber	trace
Sodium	140 mg
Magnesium	10 mg

4. Spread bread generously with Almond Pesto; arrange on prepared baking sheet.
5. Using scissors, cut sun-dried tomatoes into 1-inch (2.5 cm) pieces. Put 1 piece sun-dried tomato on each slice of bread. Sprinkle with mozzarella. (Pesto Croustades may be assembled to this point, left on baking sheet, covered, and frozen for up to 2 months.)
6. Bake room-temperature or frozen croustades in 375°F (190°C) oven for 5 to 7 minutes or until heated through and cheese has melted. Serve immediately.

Salmon Dip or Spread

Makes 1 1/2 cups (375 mL)

This is one recipe that can be used many ways. Remember that basic black dress? The one that will take you anywhere? This recipe shares that versatile quality. The Salmon Dip or Spread can be served as is with vegetables. Or spread it on tortillas and slice into mini-sandwiches (Salmon Tortilla Roll-ups, p. 57). For a glamorous display, unmold the spread from a flan pan and garnish as a savory smoked salmon gâteau (Salmon Flan, p. 58). Whatever you decide, this recipe provides a base that is tasty and quick! You can serve the spread with small Chinese cabbage leaves for extra calcium.

1	**can (7 1/2 oz/213 g) salmon**	**1**
8 oz	**light cream cheese**	**250 g**
2 tbsp	**chopped green onion**	**25 mL**
2 tbsp	**minced fresh dill**	**25 mL**
2 tbsp	**lemon juice**	**25 mL**
1/4 tsp	**freshly ground pepper**	**1 mL**

1. Drain salmon. Remove skin. Put salmon, including bones, into bowl of food processor.
2. Add cream cheese, green onion, dill, lemon juice and pepper to food processor. Process until smooth.

VARIATION:
To make Smoked Salmon Dip or Spread, add 4 oz (125 g) shredded smoked salmon to ingredients above and process until smooth. Makes 2 cups (500 mL).

Per 2 tbsp (25 mL)	
CALCIUM	54 mg
VITAMIN D	70 IU
Calories	73
Protein	5 g
Fat	6 g
Carbohydrate	1 g
Dietary Fiber	0 g
Sodium	151 mg
Magnesium	4 mg

Salmon Tortilla Roll-Ups

A variation on a salmon sandwich, these roll-ups are great served whole for lunch or cut into pieces, as described here, for appetizers or afternoon tea. For the convenience of advance preparation, make the rolls ahead of time and wrap them tightly in plastic wrap, refrigerating for up to 1 day; at serving time, unwrap and slice.

Makes 30 pieces

1 1/2 cups	**Salmon Dip or Spread (opposite)**	**375 mL**
6	**10-inch (25 cm) flour tortillas (burrito-size)**	**6**
6	**green onions, whole**	**6**
	Lemon wedges	
	Dill sprigs	

1. Spread each tortilla with about 1/4 cup (50 mL) salmon dip.
2. Place 1 green onion at the end of each tortilla; roll up.
3. Cut each roll on the diagonal into 5 pieces. Place on serving platter garnished with lemon wedges and dill sprigs.

Per piece	
CALCIUM	41 mg
VITAMIN D	28 IU
Calories	66
Protein	3 g
Fat	3 g
Carbohydrate	7 g
Dietary Fiber	trace
Sodium	104 mg
Magnesium	5 mg

Salmon Flan

Makes about 2 cups (500 mL)

This is simple to make but impressive in looks and taste! It follows the basics of the Salmon Dip or Spread (p. 56). Serve the flan with thinly sliced rye bread or crackers.

If possible, buy smoked salmon pieces for this recipe because they are less expensive than the slices and will be pureed.

FLAN:

1	can (7 1/2 oz/213 g) salmon	1
8 oz	light cream cheese	250 g
4 oz	smoked salmon, shredded	125 g
1/4 cup	minced fresh dill	50 mL
2 tbsp	chopped green onion	25 mL
1/4 tsp	freshly ground pepper	1 mL
Pinch	cayenne pepper	Pinch
1/4 cup	lemon juice	50 mL
2 tbsp	water	25 mL
1	envelope (7 g) unflavored gelatin	1

GARNISH:

1 cup	light sour cream or drained yogurt	250 mL
Half	English cucumber, thinly sliced and cut in halves	Half
4	green onions, chopped	4
Half	sweet red pepper, chopped	Half
1/2 cup	dill sprigs	125 mL
2	hard-cooked eggs, chopped	2

1. Flan: Line 8-inch (20 cm) flan pan, springform pan or cake pan with plastic wrap.
2. Drain salmon. Remove skin. Put salmon, including bones, in bowl of food processor.
3. Add cream cheese, smoked salmon, dill, green onion, pepper and cayenne pepper. Process until smooth. Keep salmon mixture in processor bowl.

Per 2 tbsp (25 mL), without garnish

CALCIUM	42 mg
VITAMIN D	52 IU
Calories	65
Protein	5 g
Fat	5 g
Carbohydrate	1 g
Dietary Fiber	0 g
Sodium	169 mg
Magnesium	5 mg

4. In small saucepan, combine lemon juice and water. Stir in gelatin. Over medium heat, stir until gelatin dissolves and mixture clears, about 2 minutes.
5. With food processor running, pour gelatin mixture through feed tube, processing until smoothly combined with salmon mixture.
6. Spoon mixture into prepared pan, leveling top. Cover with plastic wrap. Refrigerate until set, about 2 hours. Remove plastic covering. Invert flan onto serving platter. Remove flan pan and discard plastic wrap.
7. Garnish: Spread top of flan with sour cream. Arrange cucumber slices around outside base of flan to create scalloped edge. On top of flan, starting from outside edge to inside, arrange rows of green onions, then red pepper, dill sprigs and finally circle of eggs in center. The top should be completely covered.

Open-Face Sardine Sandwiches

Makes 4 servings

Reminiscent of a Scandinavian smorgasbord, these mouth-watering open-face sandwiches are a source of calcium. The sardine bones are an excellent source of calcium, so leave them in. Serve these finger sandwiches for lunch, afternoon tea or as a snack.

1	**can (3 3/4 oz/106 g) sardines packed in water**	**1**
4	**slices multigrain bread**	**4**
	Butter, softened	
1	**small red onion, thinly sliced**	**1**
	Fresh dill sprigs	

1. Drain sardines; pat dry on paper towels. Separate each sardine into two fillets. Cut each fillet in half.
2. Toast bread; trim crusts. Cut toast into neat fingers; lightly butter.
3. Divide sardine pieces among toast slices. Top with sliced red onion; sprinkle with dill.

Per serving	
CALCIUM	118 mg
VITAMIN D	38 IU
Calories	159
Protein	7 g
Fat	7 g
Carbohydrate	18 g
Dietary Fiber	2 g
Sodium	266 mg
Magnesium	17 mg

Spiced Almonds

You can never make enough of these tantalizing treats. Look for five-spice powder in the gourmet section of supermarkets and Oriental markets.

Makes 1 1/2 cups (375 mL)

1/4 cup	**granulated sugar**	**50 mL**
1 tbsp	**vegetable oil**	**15 mL**
1 tbsp	**water**	**15 mL**
1 1/2 cups	**whole unblanched almonds**	**375 mL**
2 tsp	**five-spice powder***	**10 mL**
1/4 tsp	**salt**	**1 mL**

1. Preheat oven to 350°F (180°C). Spray baking sheet with nonstick cooking spray.
2. In saucepan, bring sugar, oil and water to boil. Remove from heat. Stir in almonds, five-spice powder and salt, coating evenly.
3. Spread almonds onto prepared baking sheet.
4. Bake in 350°F (180°C) oven for 20 minutes, stirring occasionally. Spiced Almonds keep well for up to 2 days at room temperature. For longer storage, pack in plastic containers and freeze for up to 2 months.

***Chinese five-spice powder is a mixture of fennel, cloves, star anise, cinnamon and pepper.**

Per 2 tbsp (25 mL)	
CALCIUM	51 mg
Calories	132
Protein	4 g
Fat	10 g
Carbohydrate	8 g
Dietary Fiber	1 g
Sodium	50 mg
Magnesium	53 mg

Savory Munch

Makes 5 cups (1.25 L)

A sophisticated nibble with calcium crunch, this is addictive!

2 cups	mini-shredded wheat squares	500 mL
2 cups	toasted oat cereal rounds	500 mL
1 cup	whole almonds	250 mL
1/4 cup	shelled salted sunflower seeds	50 mL
1/2 tsp	salt	2 mL
1/2 tsp	dried basil	2 mL
1/2 tsp	dried rosemary	2 mL
2 tbsp	vegetable oil	25 mL
2	cloves garlic, minced	2

1. Preheat oven to 350°F (180°C). Grease baking sheet or spray with nonstick cooking spray.
2. In bowl, combine mini-shredded squares, toasted oat cereal rounds, almonds, sunflower seeds, salt, basil and rosemary.
3. In saucepan, heat oil over medium heat. Add garlic; cook, stirring, for 1 minute. Pour oil over cereal mixture, stirring to combine. Spread mixture onto prepared baking sheet.
4. Bake in 350°F (180°C) oven for 20 minutes, stirring occasionally. Store in a glass jar or a cookie tin for up to a week. It can be frozen for longer storage.

Per 1/2 cup (125 mL)	
CALCIUM	55 mg
Calories	182
Protein	5 g
Fat	12 g
Carbohydrate	16 g
Dietary Fiber	3 g
Sodium	267 mg
Magnesium	61 mg

Sweet Munch

A batch of this calcium treat won't last long. It is a tasty snack packed in a lunch, or munch on some while watching television. Make sure to serve it in small batches and hide the rest!

Makes 5 cups (1.25 L)

4 cups	**mixed cereal (mini-shredded wheat squares, toasted oat cereal rounds and other favorite cereals)**	**1 L**
1 cup	**whole almonds**	**250 mL**
1/4 cup	**sesame seeds**	**50 mL**
2 tsp	**cinnamon**	**10 mL**
1/2 cup	**packed brown sugar**	**125 mL**
1/4 cup	**butter**	**50 mL**
1/4 cup	**molasses**	**50 mL**

1. Preheat oven to 350°F (180°C). Spray baking sheet with nonstick cooking spray.
2. In bowl, combine cereal, almonds, sesame seeds and cinnamon.
3. In large saucepan, bring brown sugar, butter and molasses to boil. Remove from heat. Add cereal mixture; stir to combine. Spread mixture onto prepared sheet.
4. Bake in 350°F (180°C) oven for 20 minutes, stirring occasionally. Store in a glass jar or a cookie tin for up to a week. It can be frozen for longer storage.

Per 1/2 cup (125 mL)	
CALCIUM	84 mg
Calories	264
Protein	5 g
Fat	14 g
Carbohydrate	32 g
Dietary Fiber	3 g
Sodium	181 mg
Magnesium	76 mg

Sardine Tapenade

Makes 1 cup (250 mL)

A full-bodied Mediterranean-style calcium spread, this goes well with sliced baguette or melba toast. Garnish with lemon slices, chopped green onions and sliced olives.

1	**can (3 3/4 oz/106 g) sardines, drained**	**1**
1 cup	**sliced black olives**	**250 mL**
1/2 cup	**chopped fresh parsley**	**125 mL**
2 tbsp	**olive oil**	**25 mL**
2 tbsp	**lemon juice**	**25 mL**
1 tsp	**drained capers**	**5 mL**
2	**cloves garlic, minced**	**2**

1. Pat sardines dry on paper towel.
2. In food processor, combine sardines including bones, olives, parsley, olive oil, lemon juice, capers and garlic, processing until almost smooth.
3. Spoon spread into serving dish. Tapenade should be made and served the same day.

Per 2 tbsp (25 mL)	
CALCIUM	63 mg
VITAMIN D	19 IU
Calories	69
Protein	3 g
Fat	6 g
Carbohydrate	2 g
Dietary Fiber	1 g
Sodium	195 mg
Magnesium	8 mg

Fruit and Noodle Casserole (page 20)
with Mocaccino (page 36)
(*Overleaf*) Broccoli-Feta Soufflé (page 114),
Mediterranean Bean Salad (page 79) and
Oriental Coleslaw (page 82)

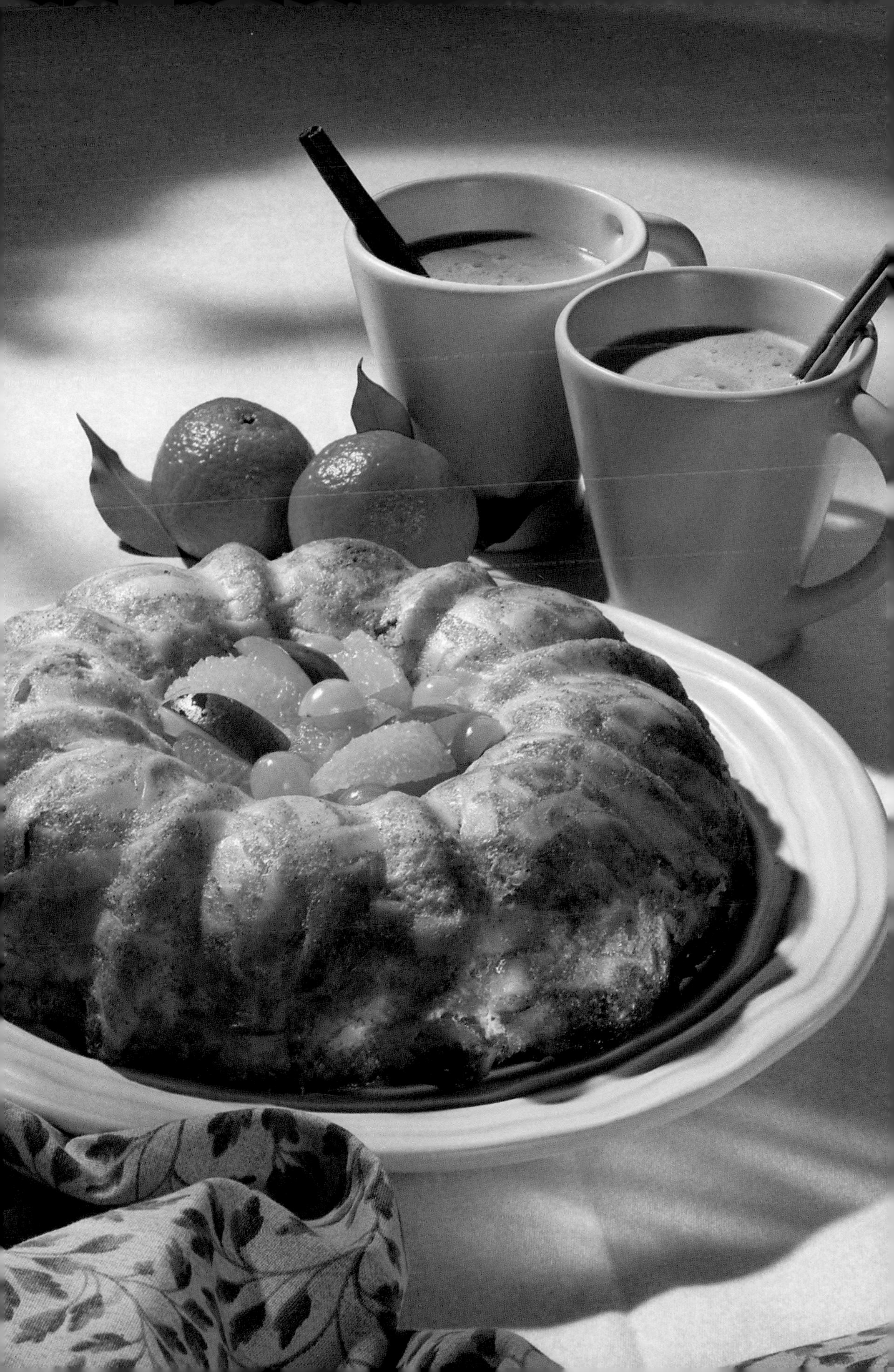

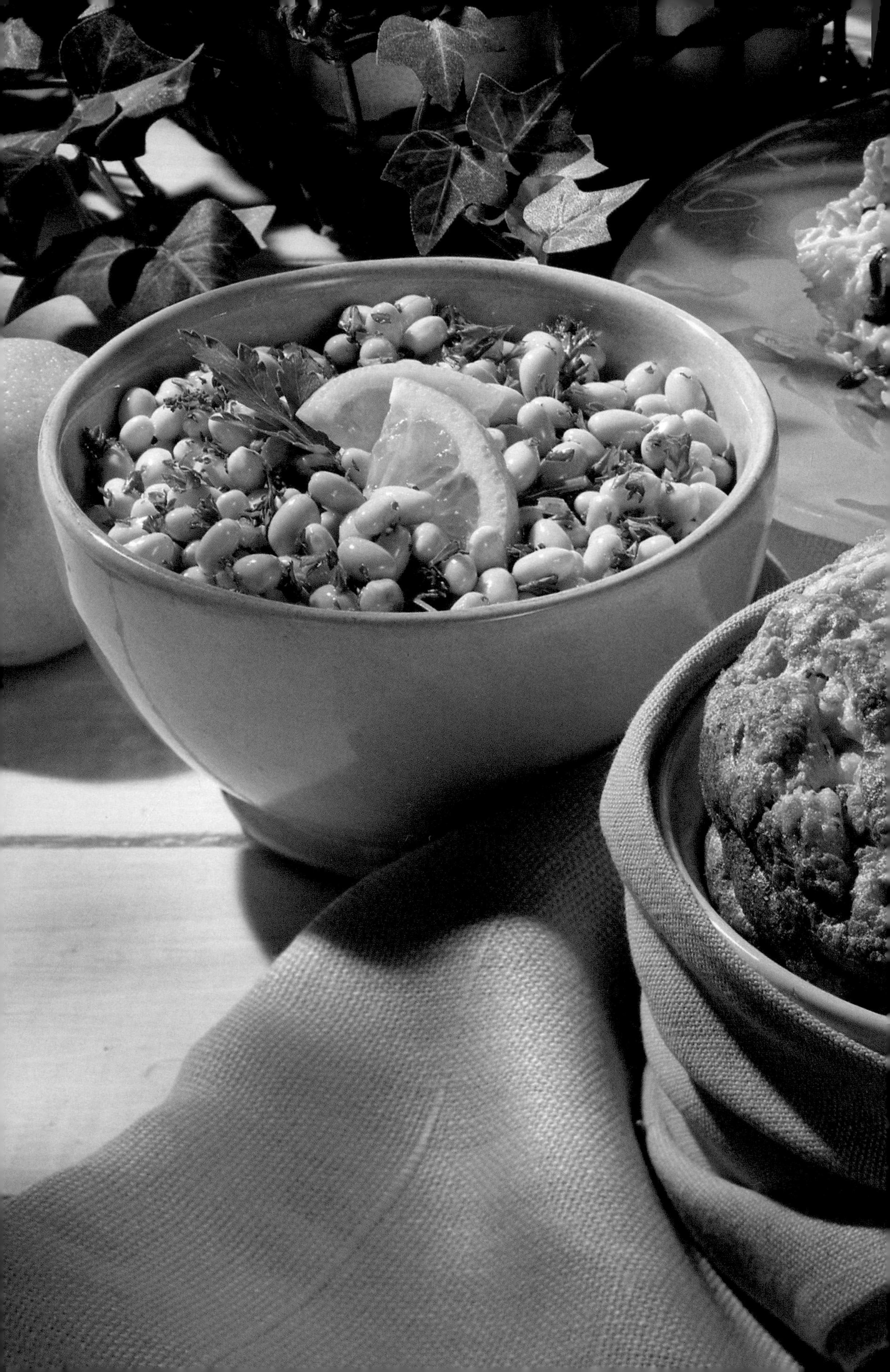

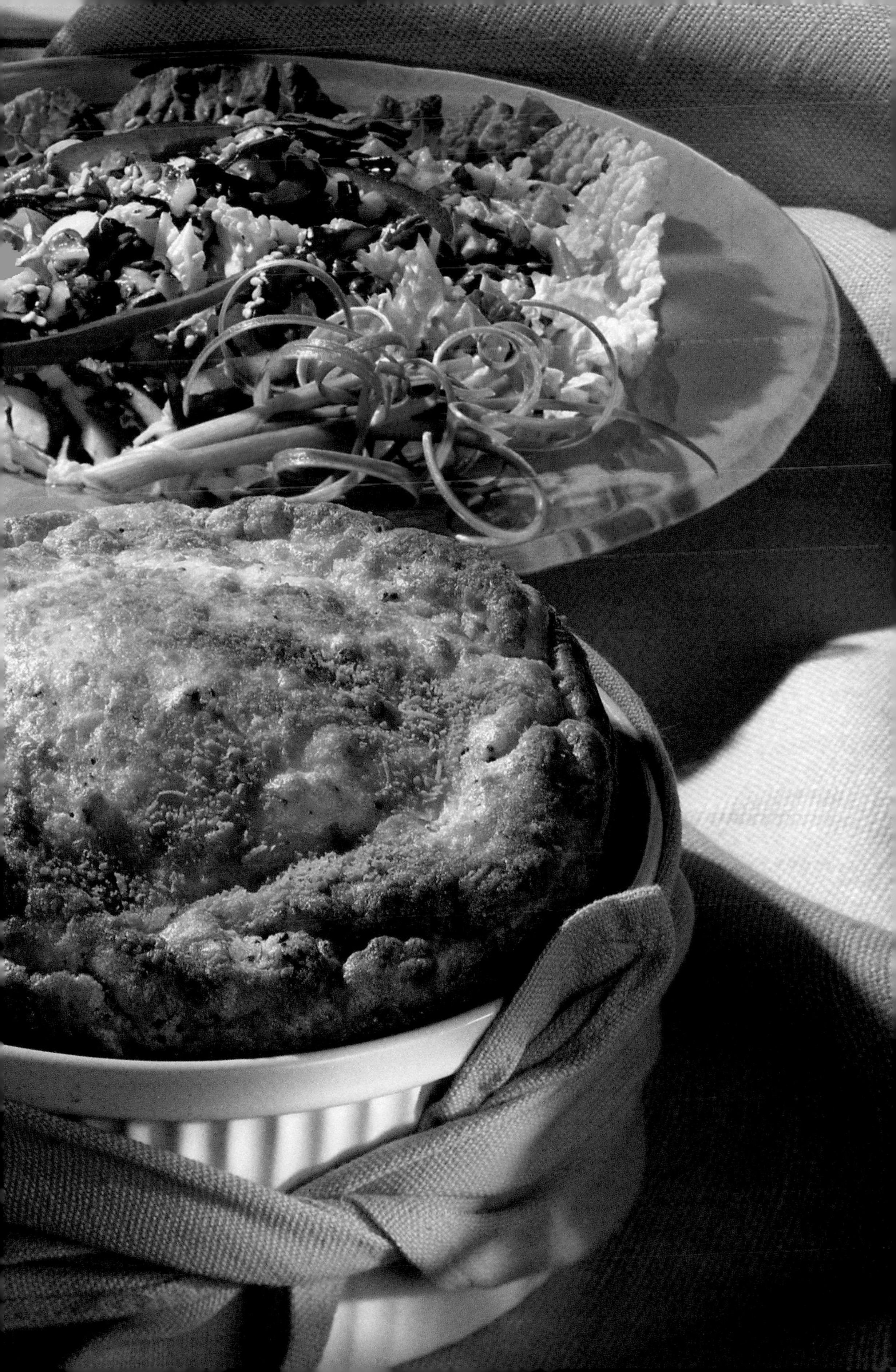

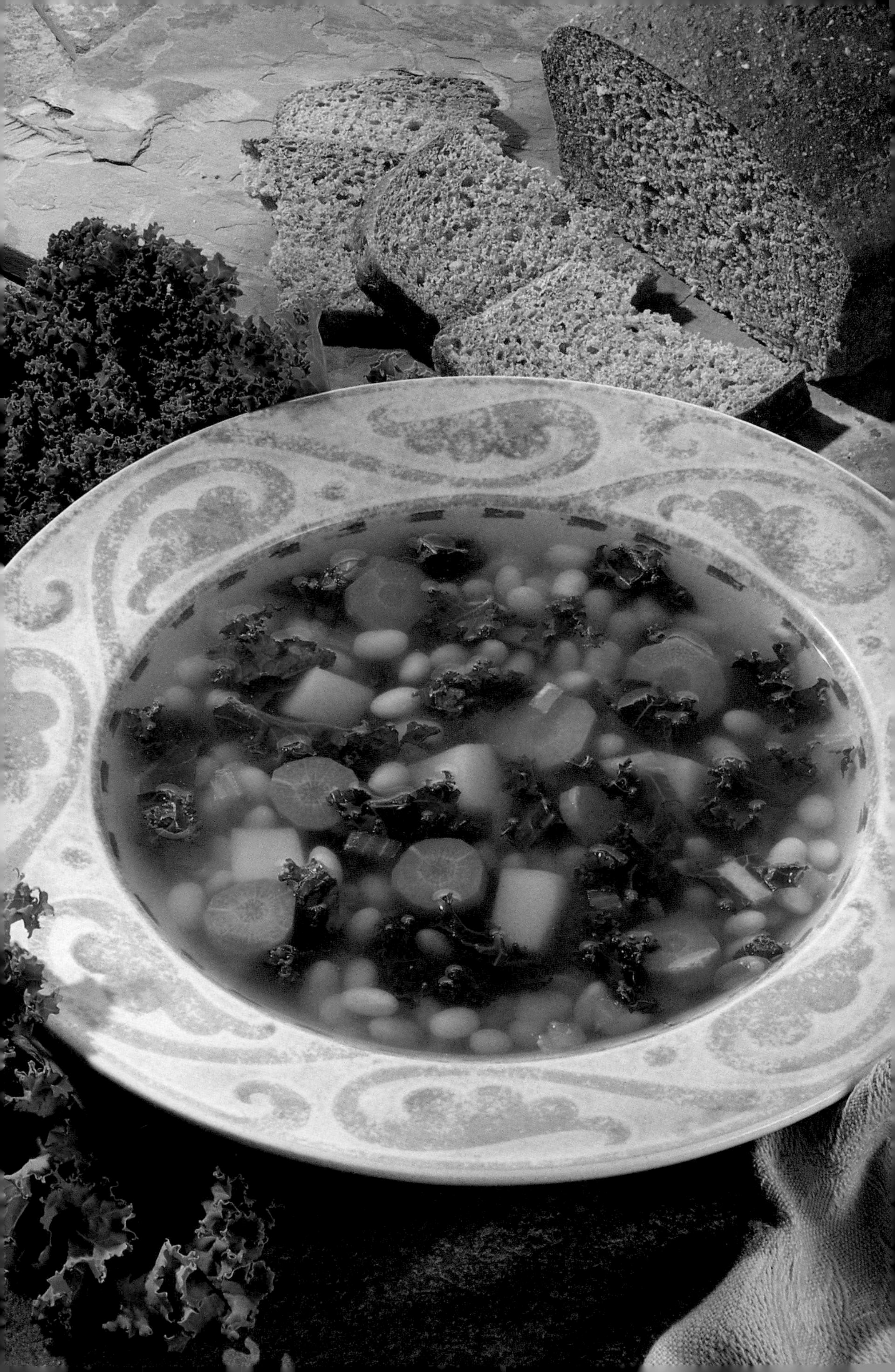

Chapter 5

Soups

Soups provide a great way to incorporate stocks made from bones, which are rich in calcium. If you don't have the time to make your own stock, then use reduced-salt canned broth. The Osteoporosis Society of Canada rccommends keeping salt intake to a minimum. Of course, ingredients containing calcium, such as beans, kale, tofu or shellfish, will give extra flavor and variety in texture when added to soups. Or, make your soup creamy and boost the calcium content at the same time by using evaporated milk, which gives the consistency of whipping cream but with much less fat. Try yogurt or light sour cream as other alternatives. Don't forget to add a calcium garnish of toasted almonds or sesame seeds.

Bean-Kale Soup (page 70) with
Whole Wheat Calcium-Yeast Bread (page 30)

Turkey Stock Using Carcass

Makes about 12 cups (3 L)

Don't throw out that turkey carcass! You have the basis of a hearty soup bursting with good taste and calcium. Many people complain that their stock lacks flavor. The reason can be that too much water and not enough vegetables and herbs have been added to create a rich-tasting stock. You won't be disappointed with this one.

Freeze stock in convenient 1-cup (250 mL) or 2-cup (500 mL) amounts.

6	whole cloves	6
1	onion	1
1	turkey carcass	1
12 to 14 cups	(approx) cold water	3 to 3.5 L
2	carrots, chopped	2
2	stalks celery, chopped	2
2 tbsp	fresh lemon juice	25 mL
6	whole peppercorns	6
4	sprigs parsley	4
1	bay leaf	1
1 tsp	thyme	5 mL

1. Push cloves into onion.
2. In large saucepan, place carcass (broken up), enough cold water to cover, onion stuck with cloves, carrots, celery, lemon juice, peppercorns, parsley, bay leaf and thyme.
3. Bring to boil. Reduce heat; simmer, uncovered, for 1 1/2 hours. Let cool.
4. Set fine sieve over large container. Ladle stock into sieve, leaving behind dregs. Strip any meat from bones; reserve meat for Turkey Soup (p. 68). Discard bay leaf, bones and vegetables. Let stock cool; remove any fat congealed on surface.

Turkey or Chicken Stock Using Necks

Make a batch of this flavorful stock and keep it frozen in usable quantities ready to add to soups, stews or casseroles. Turkey stock provides some calcium, which is leeched from the bones during the cooking process.

Makes about 15 cups (3.75 L)

3 1/2 lb	turkey or chicken necks	1.75 kg
2 tbsp	fresh lemon juice	25 mL
1	carrot	1
1	stalk celery	1
1	onion	1
3	sprigs fresh parsley	3
3	cloves garlic, cut in half	3
2	bay leaves	2
1/2 tsp	whole black peppercorns	2 mL
1/2 tsp	dried thyme	2 mL
1 tbsp	salt	15 mL

Turkey or chicken backs, wings and carcass can all be used to make stock.

1. Rinse turkey necks; place necks in 26-cup (6.5 L) stockpot. Add lemon juice, carrot, celery, onion, parsley, garlic, bay leaves, peppercorns and thyme. Add enough cold water to cover.
2. Bring to boil over high heat, skimming any scum that arises. Reduce heat; simmer, uncovered, for 1 1/2 hours.
3. Turn heat off. Set fine sieve over large bowl or container. Ladle stock into sieve, leaving dregs behind. (Do not pour all stockpot contents into sieve.) Remove necks; reserve meat for another use.
4. Stir salt into hot, strained stock. Pour into 2-cup (500 mL) and 4-cup (1 L) plastic containers. Cover and refrigerate. Once chilled, skim off any fat. Stock will keep for up to 3 months in freezer.

Turkey Soup

Makes about 12 cups (3 L)

This is easy and quick to make if you already have some de-fatted reserved turkey stock in the freezer.

12 cups	**(approx) Turkey Stock Using Carcass (p. 66)**	**3 L**
2	**carrots, chopped**	**2**
2	**stalks celery, chopped**	**2**
1	**onion or leek, chopped**	**1**
1/2 cup	**uncooked small pasta shapes or rice**	**125 mL**
	Reserved turkey meat (from Turkey Stock Using Carcass, p. 66)	
1/2 cup	**chopped fresh parsley**	**125 mL**
1 tsp	**salt**	**5 mL**
	Freshly ground black pepper	

1. In stockpot, combine turkey stock, carrots, celery, onion and pasta. Bring to boil. Reduce heat; simmer until vegetables are tender, about 20 minutes.
2. Stir in turkey meat and parsley. Season with salt and pepper to taste. Serve immediately. Any left-over soup may be covered and frozen for up to 1 month.

Per 1 1/2 cups (375 mL)	
CALCIUM	39 mg
Calories	153
Protein	17 g
Fat	3 g
Carbohydrate	12 g
Dietary Fiber	1 g
Sodium	366 mg
Magnesium	23 mg

Asparagus Tarragon Soup

This is springtime heaven in a bowl! Make it at the peak of asparagus season and serve it with a garnish of softly whipped cream, if you dare, and blanched asparagus tips.

Makes 5 cups (1.25 L), 4 servings

3 1/2 cups	chicken stock or turkey stock (preferably homemade)	875 mL
1 lb	trimmed asparagus, cut into 1-inch (2.5 cm) lengths	500 g
1/4 cup	white wine	50 mL
1 tbsp	chopped fresh tarragon	15 mL
2 tbsp	butter	25 mL
2 tbsp	all-purpose flour	25 mL
1	can (385 mL) 2% evaporated milk	1
	Salt	
	Freshly ground black pepper	
	Asparagus tips	

To get 1 lb (500 g) trimmed asparagus, you will need to buy 2 lb (1 kg).

1. In large saucepan, bring stock to boil. Reserving a few tips for garnish, add the asparagus. Reduce heat; simmer, covered, for 15 minutes or until asparagus is very tender. Transfer asparagus and stock to blender.
2. In small saucepan, bring wine to boil. Add tarragon; continue boiling until liquid has been reduced by half.
3. Add wine mixture to asparagus mixture in blender. Purée until smooth.
4. In large saucepan, melt butter over medium heat. Add flour; cook, stirring, for about 8 minutes or until golden brown. Remove from heat.
5. Gradually whisk asparagus purée into flour mixture. Return to heat; cook, stirring, until thickened.
6. Transfer asparagus purée to blender. Add milk; purée until smooth. Season with salt and pepper to taste. Pour into serving bowls. Garnish with asparagus tips.

Per serving	
CALCIUM	322 mg
VITAMIN D	76 IU
Calories	226
Protein	15 g
Fat	9 g
Carbohydrate	20 g
Dietary Fiber	2 g
Sodium	617 mg
Magnesium	42 mg

Bean-Kale Soup

Makes 8 cups (2 L), 4 servings

Here's a hearty soup to chase the chills away and make your bones stronger, too! Navy beans (or soybeans), kale and homemade chicken stock (or turkey stock) all provide calcium.

BEANS:

1 cup	dried navy (pea) beans	250 mL
1	whole clove	1
1	onion	1
1	carrot	1
1	stalk celery	1
1	bay leaf	1
1	clove garlic, cut in half	1

SOUP:

4 cups	coarsely chopped kale (stems removed)	1 L
2 tbsp	olive oil	25 mL
1 cup	chopped onion	250 mL
2	cloves garlic, minced	2
2	potatoes, peeled and chopped (about 1/2 lb/250 g)	2
1 cup	chopped carrots	250 mL
4 cups	chicken or turkey stock (preferably homemade)	1 L
1 tsp	salt	5 mL
1/4 tsp	pepper	1 mL
1 tbsp	lemon juice	15 mL

1. Beans: Rinse beans; put in saucepan with 3 cups (750 mL) water. Bring to boil. Cook at full boil for 10 minutes. Turn heat off; cover and let stand for 1 hour. Drain beans. Return beans to saucepan.

To cut down on the time of rehydrating the dried navy beans, you can simply rinse and drain 1 can (19 oz/540 mL) soybeans or canned navy beans available in some supermarkets and proceed directly to the soup section of the recipe.

Per serving	
CALCIUM	178 mg
Calories	375
Protein	18 g
Fat	9 g
Carbohydrate	56 g
Dietary Fiber	13 g
Sodium	1114 mg
Magnesium	107 mg

2. Push clove into onion; add onion to beans in saucepan. Add carrot, celery, bay leaf and garlic; add enough cold water to cover. Bring to boil. Reduce heat; simmer, covered, for 45 minutes. Check beans for tenderness and continue cooking for 15 minutes or longer or until beans are tender. Drain beans; remove and discard the bay leaf and seasoning vegetables.
3. Soup: In large pot of boiling water, cook kale for 5 minutes. Drain in colander, rinse with cold water and press to remove excess moisture.
4. In large saucepan, heat olive oil over medium heat. Add onion and garlic; cook for about 2 minutes or until onion is softened.
5. Stir in potatoes, carrots and kale; cook for 4 minutes. Pour in stock. Stir in beans, salt and pepper. Cook, covered, for 10 minutes or until vegetables are soft. Remove from heat; stir in lemon juice.

Corn Chowder

Makes 9 cups (2.25 L), about 6 servings

This is comfort food at its best. While I was growing up, this soup was made every winter from my grandmother's recipe. My mother prepared it as the main course and served it with hearty bread and a substantial pudding to follow. We loved it. I continue to make it for my own family and serve it with the Whole Wheat Calcium-Yeast Bread (p. 30) and Any-Fruit Crisp (p. 158).

2	large carrots	2
1	large onion	1
1	potato	1
1/4 cup	pearl barley	50 mL
1	can (14 oz/398 mL) creamed corn	1
1	can (385 mL) 2% evaporated milk	1
1 tsp	salt	5 mL
1/4 tsp	pepper	1 mL

1. Peel and coarsely chop carrots, onion and potato. Put in food processor; process until finely chopped.
2. Put carrot mixture and barley in large saucepan; add enough cold water to cover. Bring to boil. Reduce heat to medium; cook, covered, for 40 to 45 minutes or until barley is tender.
3. Stir in corn, milk, salt and pepper. Cook over medium-low heat, stirring frequently, until heated through. Taste and adjust seasoning if necessary.

Per serving	
CALCIUM	321 mg
VITAMIN D	76 IU
Calories	280
Protein	12 g
Fat	3 g
Carbohydrate	56 g
Dietary Fiber	6 g
Sodium	1030 mg
Magnesium	69 mg

Sweet Potato Vichyssoise

Thanks to the texture of the sweet potato, this soup is rich and velvety without cream! For those who prefer a hot soup, this rendition is equally delicious hot or cold. The evaporated milk is a concentrated calcium source.

Makes about 10 cups (2.5 L), 8 servings

2 tbsp	butter	25 mL
2	leeks, chopped	2
2 lb	sweet potatoes (about 2), peeled and chopped	1 kg
5 cups	chicken stock	1.25 L
1	bay leaf	1
1/4 tsp	curry powder	1 mL
2 cups	2% evaporated milk	500 mL
1/2 tsp	salt	2 mL
1/4 tsp	black pepper	1 mL
	Chopped chives or green onions	

1. In large saucepan over medium-high heat, melt butter.
2. Add leeks; cook, covered, for about 5 minutes or until tender. Add potatoes, stock, bay leaf and curry powder; bring to boil. Reduce heat; cook, covered, for about 20 minutes or until potatoes are tender.
3. Discard bay leaf. Using blender or food processor, purée potato mixture in batches. Stir in milk, salt and pepper. Vichyssoise may be kept covered and refrigerated for up to 2 days. When serving, garnish with sprinkling of chives.

Per serving	
CALCIUM	218 mg
VITAMIN D	47 IU
Calories	202
Protein	9 g
Fat	5 g
Carbohydrate	30 g
Dietary Fiber	3 g
Sodium	561 mg
Magnesium	39 mg

Chunky Vegetable Minestrone

Makes 8 cups (2 L), 4 servings

This hearty soup-stew made with soybeans and homemade stock helps build strong bones. Canned soybeans are available in many supermarkets and health food stores. Serve this minestrone with Focaccia *(p. 98)* *or crusty bread for a sustaining lunch or supper on a chilly day.*

4 cups	coarsely chopped kale (stems removed)	1 L
1 tbsp	olive oil	15 mL
1 cup	chopped onion	250 mL
2	carrots, chopped	2
2	stalks celery, chopped	2
1	clove garlic, minced	1
1	can (28 oz/796 mL) chopped tomatoes	1
1	can (19 oz/540 mL) soybeans, drained and rinsed	1
2 cups	turkey stock or chicken stock	500 mL
1/2 tsp	dried basil	2 mL
1/2 tsp	dried oregano	2 mL
1	bay leaf	1
Dash	hot pepper sauce	Dash
	Salt	
	Pepper	
	Freshly grated Parmesan cheese (optional)	

1. In large pot of boiling water, cook kale for 5 minutes. Drain in colander; rinse with cold water. Press to remove excess moisture.
2. In large saucepan, heat olive oil over medium heat. Add onion, carrots, celery and garlic; cook, covered, for about 5 minutes or until onion is softened. Pour in 1/4 cup (50 mL) water if vegetables begin to stick.
3. Stir in kale, tomatoes with juice, beans, stock, basil, oregano and bay leaf. Cook, covered, for 20 to 25 minutes or until vegetables are tender.

Per serving	
CALCIUM	197 mg
Calories	243
Protein	16 g
Fat	10 g
Carbohydrate	27 g
Dietary Fiber	8 g
Sodium	940 mg
Magnesium	96 mg

4. Discard bay leaf. Add hot pepper sauce. Season with salt and pepper to taste. Ladle into serving bowls. Sprinkle with Parmesan cheese (if using).

VARIATION:
Instead of the canned soybeans, you may use 1 1/2 cups (375 mL) cooked navy (pea) beans. Refer to Best Beans (p. 111) for cooking instructions for dried navy beans.

Blender Curried-Shrimp Soup

When the lazy, hazy hot days of summer arrive, this is the calcium-enhanced soup to whip up in minutes. Serve with tzatziki (a variation of Cucumber-Dill Sauce, p. 44) and Tortilla Crisps (p. 53).

Makes 2 servings

A blender always gives a smoother texture to a soup than does a food processor.

1	can (4 oz/113 g) baby shrimp	1
1 cup	buttermilk	250 mL
1/4 cup	light sour cream	50 mL
1 tbsp	minced green onion	15 mL
3/4 tsp	curry powder	4 mL

1. Drain and rinse shrimp. In blender, combine shrimp, buttermilk, sour cream, green onion and curry powder; purée until smooth. Serve chilled.

Per serving	
CALCIUM	240 mg
Calories	155
Protein	19 g
Fat	4 g
Carbohydrate	10 g
Dietary Fiber	trace
Sodium	251 mg
Magnesium	39 mg

Cucumber-Yogurt Soup

Makes 4 cups (1 L), 4 servings

Contribute to your calcium requirements with this refreshing summer soup. Yogurt, evaporated milk and almonds contribute calcium to this super-simple soup—the answer to easy summer living. Serve with Salmon and New Potato Salad (p. 84) and Whole Wheat Calcium-Yeast Bread (p. 30).

1	English cucumber	1
2 cups	1% plain yogurt	500 mL
1 cup	2% evaporated milk	250 mL
2 tbsp	minced fresh mint	25 mL
4 tsp	lemon juice	20 mL
1	clove garlic, minced	1
1/2 tsp	salt	2 mL
	Pepper	
	Toasted chopped almonds	

1. Grate cucumber. Drain in colander, pressing to remove excess moisture.
2. In bowl, stir together cucumber, yogurt, evaporated milk, mint, lemon juice, garlic, salt and pepper to taste.
3. Serve garnished with chopped almonds.

Per serving	
CALCIUM	410 mg
VITAMIN D	55 IU
Calories	144
Protein	12 g
Fat	3 g
Carbohydrate	19 g
Dietary Fiber	1 g
Sodium	446 mg
Magnesium	47 mg

Chapter 6

Salads and Salad Dressings

There are numerous ways to raise the calcium level in salads—by the innovative choice of ingredients and the choice of dressings. Take an old favorite like Caesar salad and give it a new calcium-enriched face by substituting broccoli for romaine lettuce. Likewise, with a tossed green salad, make sure you add some kale and Chinese cabbage leaves to increase the calcium level. Add orange slices, almonds, sesame seeds, seafood or beans and you have boosted the calcium even more.

Salad dressings can be a source of calcium, too. They can be creamy, lower in fat and rich in calcium if you use tofu or yogurt instead of heavy-duty mayonnaise.

The recipes included here are a sampling of the many possibilities you can create for calcium-rich salads suitable for appetizers or main courses.

Sardine Apple Salad

Makes 1 1/2 cups (375 mL), 3 servings

Vibrant in taste and color, this salad is delicious served on a bed of assorted greens that have been tossed with Tarragon Vinaigrette (p. 88). Or serve the salad as a sandwich filling on a multigrain roll. Remember to include the sardine bones as a source of calcium.

1	can (3 3/4 oz/106 g) sardines packed in water	1
Half	apple, cored and chopped	Half
3 tbsp	minced red onion	50 mL
2 tbsp	minced celery	25 mL

DRESSING:

3 tbsp	light sour cream	50 mL
2 tbsp	1% plain yogurt	25 mL
1 tbsp	minced fresh dill	15 mL
1 tbsp	lemon juice	15 mL
	Salt	
	Freshly ground black pepper	

1. Drain sardines; pat dry on paper towel. Chop coarsely, including bones.
2. In mixing bowl, gently combine sardines, apple, red onion and celery.
3. Dressing: In small bowl, whisk together sour cream, yogurt, dill, lemon juice and salt and pepper to taste.
4. Pour dressing over salad; gently fold together.

Per serving	
CALCIUM	170 mg
VITAMIN D	52 IU
Calories	91
Protein	8 g
Fat	4 g
Carbohydrate	7 g
Dietary Fiber	1 g
Sodium	270 mg
Magnesium	18 mg

Mediterranean Bean Salad

Serve this as part of an antipasto plate with Calcium Greens (p. 85) or as an accompaniment to grilled meat or fish.

Makes 4 cups (1 L), 8 servings

2 cups	dried navy (pea) beans	500 mL
1	clove	1
1	onion	1
1	stalk celery	1
1	carrot	1
1	bay leaf	1
2	cloves garlic, cut in half	2
1 tsp	salt	5 mL

DRESSING:

1/2 cup	olive oil	125 mL
1/4 cup	chopped fresh parsley	50 mL
3 tbsp	lemon juice	50 mL
2	cloves garlic, minced	2
1/4 tsp	salt	1 mL

1. To cook dried navy beans, rinse beans; add to large pot with 6 cups (1.5 L) water. Bring to boil. Cook at full boil for 10 minutes. Turn heat off, cover pot and let stand for 1 hour. Drain beans.
2. Push clove into onion.
3. In same pot, combine beans, onion, celery, carrot, bay leaf and garlic. Add enough cold water to cover. Bring to boil. Reduce heat; simmer, covered, for 45 minutes. Add salt; simmer for 15 minutes or until beans are tender. Drain beans; discard other ingredients.
4. Dressing: In small bowl, whisk together oil, parsley, lemon juice, garlic and salt. Pour dressing over beans; toss to coat. Serve salad warm or at room temperature.

VARIATION:

You can use 1 can (19 oz/540 mL) navy beans or soy beans that have been drained and rinsed in place of the dried navy (pea) beans and go straight to step 2.

Per serving	
CALCIUM	88 mg
Calories	289
Protein	10 g
Fat	14 g
Carbohydrate	32 g
Dietary Fiber	9 g
Sodium	352 mg
Magnesium	71 mg

Broccoli Caesar Salad

Makes 4 servings

A variation on a popular recipe, this Caesar version acquires calcium from broccoli and the dressing—whether you use the Caesar Dressing (p. 91) where the calcium sources are yogurt and anchovies or the Lactose-Free Caesar Dressing (p. 90) where the calcium sources are tofu and anchovies.

SALAD:

1	**bunch broccoli (about 6 cups/1.5 L florets and thinly sliced peeled stems)**	**1**
6 oz	**back bacon**	**170 g**

CROUTONS:

2 tbsp	**olive oil**	**25 mL**
1	**clove garlic, crushed**	**1**
4	**slices whole-grain bread or French-style loaf**	**4**

DRESSING:

Caesar Dressing (p. 91) or Lactose-Free Caesar Dressing (p. 90)

1. Salad: In saucepan of rapidly boiling water, cook broccoli, uncovered, for 3 minutes or until tender-crisp. Drain and run under cold water to stop broccoli cooking.
2. Chop bacon. Cook in frying pan over medium-high heat for 10 minutes, stirring occasionally, or until desired crispness. Drain on paper towels.
3. Croutons: Preheat oven to 350°F (180°C). Meanwhile, in small bowl, combine oil and garlic.
4. Using pastry brush, brush oil mixture lightly over both sides of bread. Trim off crusts; cut remaining bread into 1/2-inch (1 cm) cubes.
5. Bake bread cubes on baking sheet in 350°F (180°C) oven for 20 to 25 minutes or until golden brown.
6. Assembly: In serving bowl, combine broccoli, bacon bits and enough dressing to coat broccoli. Garnish with croutons.

Per serving	
CALCIUM	112 mg
Calories	254
Protein	16 g
Fat	13 g
Carbohydrate	21 g
Dietary Fiber	5 g
Sodium	896 mg
Magnesium	33 mg

Broccoli-Cauliflower Salad

This dramatic salad is great for entertaining, especially since it can be made ahead. Prepare it in the autumn when broccoli and cauliflower are abundant and inexpensive.

Makes 10 cups (2.5 L), 8 servings

1	bunch broccoli	1
1	head cauliflower	1
1/2 cup	sliced sweet red pepper	125 mL
1/2 cup	sliced black olives	125 mL
2	green onions, chopped	2
3/4 cup	Tarragon Vinaigrette (p. 88)	175 mL

1. Discard tough stem end of broccoli, reserving tender portion to peel and slice thinly. Cut head into florets. Cut cauliflower into florets.
2. In large pot of boiling water, cook broccoli, uncovered, for 3 minutes or until tender-crisp. Rinse under cold water; drain. Transfer to large bowl.
3. In large pot of boiling water, cook cauliflower, uncovered, for 4 minutes or until tender-crisp. Rinse under cold water; drain. Add to broccoli. Stir in red pepper, olives and green onions.
4. Pour vinaigrette over vegetables; toss to coat. Serve immediately. Or cover and refrigerate for up to 2 days.

Per serving	
CALCIUM	58 mg
Calories	167
Protein	3 g
Fat	15 g
Carbohydrate	8 g
Dietary Fiber	3 g
Sodium	236 mg
Magnesium	25 mg

Oriental Coleslaw

Makes about 9 cups (2.25 L), 8 servings

This is not a typical coleslaw. The combination of Oriental cabbages—nappa, bok choy and Chinese cabbage—give the salad a mild flavor and contribute calcium.

7 cups	**mixture of shredded nappa, bok choy and Chinese cabbage**	**1.75 L**
2 cups	**sliced green cabbage or red cabbage**	**500 mL**
Half	**sweet red pepper, sliced**	**Half**
4	**green onions, chopped**	**4**
1/4 cup	**toasted chopped unblanched almonds**	**50 mL**
2 tbsp	**sesame seeds**	**25 mL**

DRESSING:

1/3 cup	**vegetable oil**	**75 mL**
1/4 cup	**white wine vinegar**	**50 mL**
1 tbsp	**granulated sugar**	**15 mL**
1 tbsp	**sesame oil**	**15 mL**
1	**large clove garlic, minced**	**1**
1 tsp	**salt**	**5 mL**
1/2 tsp	**pepper**	**2 mL**

1. In large bowl, combine nappa, bok choy, Chinese cabbage, green cabbage, red pepper, green onions, almonds and sesame seeds. (Salad may be assembled to this point, covered and refrigerated for up to 1 day.)
2. Dressing: In blender, combine vegetable oil, vinegar, sugar, sesame oil, garlic, salt and pepper; purée.
3. Pour dressing over salad; toss gently to coat.

Per serving	
CALCIUM	101 mg
Calories	157
Protein	3 g
Fat	14 g
Carbohydrate	6 g
Dietary Fiber	2 g
Sodium	326 mg
Magnesium	38 mg

The Ultra-Calcium Greek Salad

Kale, nappa cabbage, Caesar dressing and feta cheese help boost the calcium content of this popular salad. Be sure to use at least 3 cups (750 mL) each of kale and nappa in the greens mixture.

Makes 2 main-course servings or 4 appetizer servings

8 cups	mixed torn greens (combination of kale, nappa cabbage and romaine)	2 L
2	tomatoes, sliced	2
1/2 cup	thinly sliced red onion	125 mL
1/2 cup	cucumber (cut into chunks)	125 mL
1/2 cup	black olives	125 mL
1/3 cup	Caesar Dressing (p. 91)	75 mL
1/2 cup	crumbled feta cheese (about 2 oz/50 g)	125 mL

1. In large mixing bowl, combine greens, tomatoes, red onion, cucumber and olives.
2. Pour dressing over vegetables; toss gently to coat.
3. Divide salad among serving plates; sprinkle with feta cheese.

Per appetizer serving	
CALCIUM	248 mg
Calories	142
Protein	7 g
Fat	7 g
Carbohydrate	16 g
Dietary Fiber	5 g
Sodium	456 mg
Magnesium	43 mg

Salmon and New Potato Salad

Makes 4 cups (1 L), 4 main-course servings

Dill Vinaigrette makes 1 cup (250mL)

Salmon and new potatoes are a springtime classic. The addition of kale adds a welcome tang and more calcium to that of the salmon.

DILL VINAIGRETTE:

1/2 cup	vegetable oil	125 mL
1/4 cup	chopped fresh dill	50 mL
1/4 cup	white wine	50 mL
1/4 cup	white wine vinegar	50 mL
1 tsp	salt	5 mL
1 tsp	Dijon mustard	5 mL
1/4 tsp	freshly ground black pepper	1 mL

SALAD:

1 lb	tiny new potatoes	500 g
1	can (7 1/2 oz/213 g) salmon	1
4 cups	kale (stems removed and kale torn into bite-size pieces)	1 L
1/4 cup	chopped green onions	50 mL

1. Dill Vinaigrette: In food processor, purée vegetable oil, dill, white wine, wine vinegar, salt, mustard and pepper until smooth. Pour into jar; set aside.
2. Salad: Scrub potatoes, leaving skins on. Steam for 15 to 20 minutes or until tender. Cut in half; transfer to bowl.
3. Drain salmon. Remove and discard skin; mash bones. Flake salmon and add with bones to potatoes.
4. Assembly: In separate bowl, toss kale with 2 tbsp (25 mL) of the vinaigrette or enough to coat kale lightly.

Per main-course serving	
CALCIUM	221 mg
VITAMIN D	209 IU
Calories	336
Protein	13 g
Fat	20 g
Carbohydrate	27 g
Dietary Fiber	4 g
Sodium	577 mg
Magnesium	60 mg

5. Pour 1/2 cup (125 mL) of the vinaigrette over potatoes and salmon; toss gently to coat.
6. Serve potatoes and salmon, warm or at room temperature, over bed of kale. Sprinkle with green onions. Remaining vinaigrette will keep, covered and refrigerated, for up to 1 week.

Calcium Greens

Every cook needs a good basic green salad, and this one has a bonus—calcium. Kale, nappa, Chinese cabbage, oranges, almonds and hazelnuts all contribute calcium.

Makes 6 servings

12 cups	**mixed torn greens (kale, spinach, nappa and Chinese cabbage)**	**3 L**
2	**oranges (skin and pith removed), sliced horizontally**	**2**
1/2 cup	**toasted slivered almonds or toasted chopped hazelnuts**	**125 mL**
1/4 cup	**sliced red onion**	**50 mL**
1/4 cup	**Tarragon Vinaigrette (p. 88)**	**50 mL**

1. In large mixing bowl, toss together mixed greens, oranges, almonds and red onion. (Salad may be assembled to this point, covered, and refrigerated for up to 1 day.)
2. Just before serving, toss salad with enough dressing to coat leaves. Serve immediately.

Per serving	
CALCIUM	193 mg
Calories	287
Protein	6 g
Fat	24 g
Carbohydrate	16 g
Dietary Fiber	4 g
Sodium	266 mg
Magnesium	86 mg

Turkey Waldorf Salad

Makes 2 main-course servings

Leftover turkey never tasted so good. Change this yummy salad with the seasons—apples in autumn and winter, peaches in summer, seedless grapes in winter and summer. Serve the salad on a bed of Calcium Greens (p. 85) along with Whole-Grain Fig Bread (p. 18) for a great combination of tastes.

2 cups	**torn cooked turkey breast (about 8 oz/250 g cooked weight)**	**500 mL**
2	**stalks celery, chopped**	**2**
2	**red apples, cored and sliced**	**2**
1/4 cup	**toasted almonds**	**50 mL**
1/2 cup	**Creamy Tarragon-Yogurt Dressing (p. 88)**	**125 mL**

1. In mixing bowl, combine turkey, celery, apples and almonds.
2. Pour dressing over salad; toss until coated. Serve immediately.

VARIATIONS:

Turkey Salad Véronique:

Substitute 2 cups (500 mL) halved seedless green and red grapes for the apples.

Curried Turkey-Peach Salad:

Substitute 2 peaches (skinned and chopped) for the apples; substitute Creamy Curry Dressing (p. 89) for Creamy Tarragon-Yogurt Dressing (p. 88).

Per serving	
CALCIUM	175 mg
Calories	495
Protein	40 g
Fat	23 g
Carbohydrate	34 g
Dietary Fiber	4 g
Sodium	929 mg
Magnesium	104 mg

Warm Kale and Red Cabbage Salad

Makes 8 appetizer servings

If you want a dining-out experience in the comfort of your own home, then try this dramatic salad. By adding marinated tofu or sautéed chicken breast (when you add the fennel and apple to the salad), you have a main course in minutes. Accompany with assorted breads and wine for a delicious evening.

1/4 cup	**vegetable oil**	**50 mL**
8 cups	**finely shredded red cabbage**	**2 L**
4 cups	**kale (stems removed and kale torn into bite-size pieces)**	**1 L**
1/4 cup	**packed brown sugar**	**50 mL**
2 tbsp	**raspberry vinegar**	**25 mL**
1/2 tsp	**salt**	**2 mL**
1/4 tsp	**black pepper**	**1 mL**
1 cup	**sliced fennel**	**250 mL**
1	**red apple, cored and thinly sliced**	**1**

1. In Dutch oven or large skillet, heat 2 tbsp (25 mL) of the vegetable oil over medium-high heat.
2. Add red cabbage and kale, stir-frying for 5 minutes or until vegetables are wilted and have given off liquid. Continue to cook until all liquid has evaporated. Meanwhile, in measuring cup, whisk together remaining oil, brown sugar, vinegar, salt and pepper until well combined.
3. Pour oil mixture over vegetables. Add fennel and apple; stir-fry until vegetables are coated and hot. Serve immediately.

Per serving	
CALCIUM	95 mg
Calories	136
Protein	2 g
Fat	7 g
Carbohydrate	18 g
Dietary Fiber	3 g
Sodium	173 mg
Magnesium	27 mg

Creamy Tarragon-Yogurt Dressing

Makes 3/4 cup (175 mL)

A perfect combination with fish or poultry, this recipe can double as a salad dressing (especially for pasta salads) and as a sauce for fish or poultry.

1/3 cup	1% plain yogurt	75 mL
1/4 cup	light mayonnaise	50 mL
1 tsp	dried tarragon	5 mL
1 tsp	granulated sugar	5 mL
1 tsp	red wine vinegar	5 mL
1/2 tsp	salt	2 mL
1/2 tsp	Dijon mustard	2 mL

1. In small bowl, whisk together yogurt, mayonnaise, tarragon, sugar, vinegar, salt and mustard until smooth.
2. Spoon into jar; cover and refrigerate for up to 3 days.

Per 2 tbsp (25 mL)	
CALCIUM	40 mg
Calories	62
Protein	1 g
Fat	5 g
Carbohydrate	4 g
Dietary Fiber	0 g
Sodium	408 mg
Magnesium	4 mg

Tarragon Vinaigrette

Makes 3/4 cup (175 mL)

This is a versatile dressing suitable for tossing with green salads and for marinating vegetables.

1/2 cup	extra virgin olive oil	125 mL
1/4 cup	white wine vinegar	50 mL
1	clove garlic, crushed	1
1 tsp	dried tarragon	5 mL
1 tsp	Dijon mustard	5 mL
1 tsp	granulated sugar	5 mL
1/2 tsp	salt	2 mL
1/4 tsp	freshly ground black pepper	1 mL

Per 2 tbsp (25 mL)	
CALCIUM	5 mg
Calories	164
Protein	trace
Fat	18 g
Carbohydrate	2 g
Dietary Fiber	0 g
Sodium	202 mg
Magnesium	3 mg

1. In food processor, purée olive oil, vinegar, garlic, tarragon, mustard, sugar, salt and pepper until smooth and well blended.
2. Pour into jar; cover and refrigerate for up to 1 week.

Creamy Curry Dressing

Try this piquant dressing on poultry, fruit or grain salads.

Makes 1/2 cup (125 mL)

1/3 cup	**1% plain yogurt**	**75 mL**
1/4 cup	**light mayonnaise**	**50 mL**
1 tsp	**curry powder**	**5 mL**
1 tsp	**granulated sugar**	**5 mL**

1. In small bowl, whisk together yogurt, mayonnaise, curry powder and sugar.
2. Spoon into jar; cover and refrigerate for up to 3 days.

Per 2 tbsp (25 mL)	
CALCIUM	39 mg
Calories	63
Protein	1 g
Fat	5 g
Carbohydrate	4 g
Dietary Fiber	0 g
Sodium	113 mg
Magnesium	5 mg

Lactose-Free Caesar Dressing

Makes about 1 1/3 cups (325 mL)

One of the most popular salad dressings, Caesar mixtures can be used as dips, as dressings for mixed greens or as pasta sauces.

1	pkg (10 1/4 oz/290 g) silken soft tofu, drained (or about 1 cup/250 mL drained)	1
7	anchovies, drained on paper towels and roughly chopped	7
2 tbsp	freshly squeezed lemon juice	25 mL
1 tbsp	vegetable oil	15 mL
2 tsp	Dijon mustard	10 mL
1/4 tsp	salt	1 mL
1/4 tsp	pepper	1 mL
Pinch	cayenne pepper	Pinch
1	clove garlic	1

1. In food processor, combine tofu, anchovies, lemon juice, oil, mustard, salt, pepper, cayenne and garlic; purée until smooth.
2. Spoon into jar; cover and refrigerate for up to two days.

Per 2 tbsp (25 mL)	
CALCIUM	24 mg
Calories	34
Protein	2 g
Fat	2 g
Carbohydrate	1 g
Dietary Fiber	0 g
Sodium	167 mg
Magnesium	2 mg

Caesar Dressing

Anchovies add zesty flavor and calcium.

Makes about 1 1/3 cups (325 mL)

1 cup	**1% plain yogurt**	**250 mL**
1/4 cup	**light mayonnaise**	**50 mL**
4	**anchovies, drained on paper towels and roughly chopped**	**4**
1 tbsp	**freshly squeezed lemon juice**	**15 mL**
1/2 tsp	**Worcestershire sauce**	**2 mL**
1/4 tsp	**salt**	**1 mL**
1	**clove garlic**	**1**
Dash	**hot sauce**	**Dash**

1. In food processor, combine yogurt, mayonnaise, anchovies, lemon juice, Worcestershire sauce, salt, garlic and hot sauce; purée until smooth.
2. Spoon into jar; cover and refrigerate for up to 4 days.

Per 2 tbsp (25 mL)	
CALCIUM	45 mg
Calories	34
Protein	2 g
Fat	2 g
Carbohydrate	2 g
Dietary Fiber	0 g
Sodium	164 mg
Magnesium	5 mg

Chapter 7

Pasta and Grains

Pasta, pizza and grains are naturals for cheese, cheese and more cheese. But not these recipes. There are a variety of other ingredients that add calcium, flavor and pizzazz. For maximum taste and a minimum of fat and lactose, use freshly grated Parmesan cheese. A little goes a long way. You also don't need heavy cheese sauces for pasta. For creamy sauces, try 2% evaporated milk instead of whipping cream for luxurious taste and silky texture. The evaporated milk provides the extra benefit of double the calcium of regular milk.

Another way to increase the calcium content of recipes is to add broccoli, kale, bok choy, Chinese cabbage, anchovies or salmon. Anchovies and salmon provide a double bonus because they contain both calcium and vitamin D. You can also make a terrific pizza crust by adding some soy flour to the mixture—more calcium with the same delectable homemade goodness and taste.

Pasta Alla Bolognese

Makes 8 servings

A welcome change from lasagna, this dish has a flavorful, calcium-rich béchamel-like sauce that is lower in fat than the usual cheese sauce. Make it ahead and serve with crusty bread and Calcium Greens (p. 85) for an easy buffet dinner.

	Turkey Sauce (p. 107)	
1 lb	fettuccine or linguine (preferably spinach pasta)	500 g

CREAM SAUCE:

1/4 cup	olive oil or butter	50 mL
1/3 cup	all-purpose flour	75 mL
6 cups	milk, soy beverage or lactose-reduced milk	1.5 L
1 tsp	grated nutmeg	5 mL
1/2 tsp	dried thyme	2 mL
1 tsp	salt	5 mL
	Freshly ground black pepper	

TOPPING:

1 cup	fresh bread crumbs (preferably whole wheat)	250 mL
1/4 cup	chopped fresh parsley	50 mL
1 tbsp	olive oil	15 mL
1/2 cup	freshly grated Parmesan cheese (optional)	125 mL

1. Grease 13- x 9-inch (3.5 L) baking dish or spray with nonstick cooking spray.
2. In large pot of boiling salted water, cook pasta for 8 to 10 minutes or until al dente. Rinse under running water; drain and set aside.

Per serving with Parmesan cheese

CALCIUM	427 mg
VITAMIN D	64 IU
Calories	611
Protein	30 g
Fat	24 g
Carbohydrate	71 g
Dietary Fiber	6 g
Sodium	1054 mg
Magnesium	167 mg

3. Cream Sauce: In saucepan, heat oil over medium-low heat. Whisk in flour. Cook, stirring, for 1 minute. Gradually add milk, whisking constantly until mixture starts to thicken. Increase heat to medium. Whisk in nutmeg, thyme, salt and pepper to taste. Cook, stirring, for 5 to 8 minutes, until thickened. Remove from heat.
4. Topping: In small bowl, combine bread crumbs, parsley and olive oil. Stir in cheese (if using).
5. Assembly: Spread half (about 3 cups/750 mL) of the Turkey Spaghetti Sauce in bottom of prepared baking dish. Top with half of the pasta; repeat layers. Spoon cream sauce evenly over top. Sprinkle evenly with topping. (Casserole may be assembled to this point, covered and refrigerated overnight; or wrap well and freeze for up to 1 month. Defrost in refrigerator overnight before baking.)
6. Bake, covered, in 375°F (190°C) oven for 30 minutes; uncover and bake for 15 minutes or until topping is golden brown.

VARIATIONS:

For a lactose-free dish, make the cream sauce with olive oil and soy beverage; and omit the cheese from the bread-crumb topping. However, this version will contain no calcium.

For more calcium, substitute 1 cup (250 mL) 2% evaporated milk for 1 cup (250 mL) of the milk in the cream sauce.

Salmon-Rice Casserole

Makes 4 servings

Salmon, dill and rice are a classic combination. This recipe has been enriched with the calcium ingredients of kale and salmon bones. Serve with Cucumber-Dill Sauce (p. 44).

1/4 cup	wild rice	50 mL
1	bay leaf	1
3/4 cup	water	175 mL
1 cup	turkey or chicken stock	250 mL
1/2 cup	parboiled long-grain white rice	125 mL
4 cups	coarsely chopped kale, stems removed	1 L
2 tbsp	butter or olive oil	25 mL
1 cup	chopped onion	250 mL
1 cup	sliced mushrooms	250 mL
1	can (7 1/2 oz/213 g) salmon	1
2	hard-cooked eggs, finely chopped	2
1/2 cup	chopped fresh parsley	125 mL
1/4 cup	chopped fresh dill	50 mL
3 tbsp	lemon juice	50 mL

Fresh kale does not keep long; use within 2 days of buying. Remove tough centre stems from leaves before using. As a guideline, 8 cups (2 L) of kale cooks down to 1 cup (250 mL).

1. Preheat oven to 350°F (180°C). Grease 6-cup (1.5 L) baking dish or spray with nonstick cooking spray.
2. In small bowl, soak wild rice for 30 minutes in enough cold water to cover. Drain.
3. In small saucepan, combine bay leaf and the 3/4 cup (175 mL) water; bring to boil. Stir in wild rice; reduce heat to medium-low. Cook, covered, for 30 minutes or until tender. Drain any excess water. Discard bay leaf.
4. In separate small saucepan, bring stock to boil. Stir in white rice; reduce heat to medium-low. Cook, covered, for 15 minutes. Remove from heat; let stand for 5 minutes.

Per serving	
CALCIUM	217 mg
VITAMIN D	227 IU
Calories	326
Protein	18 g
Fat	12 g
Carbohydrate	36 g
Dietary Fiber	4 g
Sodium	417 mg
Magnesium	58 mg

5. In large pot of boiling water, cook kale for 5 minutes. Drain in colander; rinse with cold water. Press to remove excess moisture.
6. In saucepan, melt butter over medium-high heat. Cook onion and mushrooms for 5 minutes or until tender.
7. Drain salmon. Discard skin. Flake salmon and mash bones.
8. In large bowl, combine wild rice, white rice, kale, onion-mushroom mixture, salmon (including bones), eggs, parsley, dill and lemon juice.
9. Transfer to prepared dish. Bake in 350°F (180°C) oven for 20 to 25 minutes, until heated through.

Focaccia

Makes one 12-inch (30 cm) bread, 8 wedges

Quick and easy to prepare, this Italian flatbread can be made with a variety of fresh or dried herbs. It's versatile and may be used as a base for pizza. This recipe has been enriched with calcium by the addition of skim milk powder and soy flour.

1 cup	lukewarm water	250 mL
1	pkg (8 g) traditional active dry yeast or 1 tbsp (15 mL)	1
1 tsp	granulated sugar	5 mL
3 tbsp	olive oil	50 mL
2	cloves garlic, minced	2
2 tbsp	dried herbs (mixture of rosemary, basil, sage, thyme or tarragon)	25 mL
1/2 tsp	salt	2 mL
1/2 cup	instant skim milk powder	125 mL
1 1/2 cups	(approx) all-purpose flour	375 mL
1/2 cup	soy flour or all-purpose flour	125 mL
	Cornmeal	
1 tsp	coarse salt*	5 mL

To speed up dough-rising, place bowl of dough in larger bowl of warm water. Cover dough bowl with plastic wrap. Dough will double in size in half the time.

*Coarse salt is also known as pickling salt.

1. In mixing bowl rinsed with warm water, pour in lukewarm water. Sprinkle with yeast and sugar. Let stand in warm place for 10 minutes.
2. Meanwhile, heat 2 tbsp (25 mL) of the olive oil in skillet over medium heat. Add garlic and herbs; cook, covered, until fragrant, about 30 seconds.
3. Whisk oil mixture and salt into frothy yeast. Gradually whisk in skim milk powder, enough all-purpose flour and soy flour until batter is stiff. Knead in remaining flour. If dough becomes too sticky to knead, lightly flour hands and dough. Continue to knead until dough is smooth and springy to the touch, about 5 minutes. Form into a ball.

Per wedge	
CALCIUM	82 mg
VITAMIN D	19 IU
Calories	171
Protein	7 g
Fat	6 g
Carbohydrate	24 g
Dietary Fiber	2 g
Sodium	457 mg
Magnesium	31 mg

4. Place dough in clean, oiled bowl; cover and let stand in warm place until doubled in bulk, about 1 to 1 1/2 hours.
5. Punch down dough; shape into 12-inch (30 cm) circle on pizza pan sprinkled with cornmeal. Using fingers, poke indentations into dough. Brush dough with remaining olive oil; sprinkle with coarse salt. Let rise in warm place for about 30 minutes.
6. Bake in 450°F (230°C) oven for about 20 minutes or until golden brown. Cut into wedges. Serve hot or at room temperature.

VARIATIONS:
To use this dough to make breadsticks, at Step 5, punch down dough and shape into 4 equal portions. Form each into rolls 6 inches (15 cm) long. Brush with remaining olive oil. Roll 2 of the rolls in flax seeds and the other two in sesame seeds. Taking one flax seed and one sesame seed roll, pinch ends together and twist, tucking ends under. Place on baking sheet lined with parchment paper; sprinkle dough with coarse salt. Let dough rise in warm place for about 30 minutes. Bake in 450°F (230°C) oven for about 15 minutes or until golden brown. Makes 2 large bread sticks.

You can also use baked focaccia as a base for pizza and add your favorite pizza toppings. Remember to include cheeses and anchovies as sources of calcium.

Dried or fresh herbs may be used in the recipe; if you opt for fresh herbs, use 1/4 cup (50 mL) chopped.

Asian Noodle Stir-Fry

Makes 8 cups (2 L), 4 servings

Once you have prepared the vegetables for this dish, the stir-fry can be ready in minutes. Look for Oriental supplies in the specialty section of your grocery store or in Asian supermarkets.

4 oz	rice vermicelli	125 g
1/4 cup	reduced-sodium soy sauce	50 mL
2 tbsp	rice wine for cooking (mirin)	25 mL
2 tbsp	vegetable oil	25 mL
2 tbsp	minced gingerroot	25 mL
2	cloves garlic, minced	2
2	carrots, thinly sliced on diagonal	2
1/2 lb	mushrooms, sliced	250 g
2 cups	shredded Chinese cabbage	500 mL
2 cups	shredded bok choy	500 mL
2 cups	shredded nappa cabbage	500 mL
1/4 cup	chopped fresh coriander	50 mL
1 tbsp	sesame seeds	15 mL
2	green onions, chopped	2

1. In bowl, add enough boiling water to cover vermicelli. Let stand for 15 minutes. Drain; set aside.
2. In small bowl, combine soy sauce and rice wine. Set aside.
3. In wok or large saucepan over medium-high heat, heat oil. Add ginger and garlic. Cook, stirring, for 1 minute. Add carrots and mushrooms; cook, stirring, for 6 minutes. Add Chinese cabbage, bok choy and nappa cabbage; cook, stirring, for 2 minutes or until greens wilt.
4. Stir in reserved soy sauce mixture, reserved vermicelli noodles and coriander; cook, stirring, until heated through. Remove from heat.
5. Turn out onto serving platter. Garnish with sesame seeds and green onions. Serve immediately.

VARIATION:
By adding 8 oz (250 g) sliced firm tofu or sautéed sliced chicken breast to the dish, you create a main course.

Per serving	
CALCIUM	138 mg
Calories	243
Protein	7 g
Fat	9 g
Carbohydrate	34 g
Dietary Fiber	4 g
Sodium	544 mg
Magnesium	52 mg

Calcium-Enriched Macaroni and Cheese

My teenage son devours this pasta regularly. There are no leftovers. By reducing the amount of butter called for in the recipe on the package and increasing the milk and cheese, you have a calcium-rich dish that is lower in fat. With the addition of blanched broccoli and tomato, you have a complete meal. Add zip by stirring in a spoonful of your favorite salsa.

Makes 1 teenage serving or 2 adult servings

1	**pkg (225 g) macaroni and cheese dinner**	**1**
1/2 to 1 cup	**2% milk**	**125 to 250 mL**
1/2 cup	**shredded old Cheddar cheese**	**125 mL**
1 tbsp	**butter**	**15 mL**

1. In pot of boiling water, cook macaroni for 5 to 7 minutes, until al dente. Drain.
2. Return pasta to pot; turn heat down to low.
3. Add sauce mix from box, milk, shredded cheese and butter. Cook, stirring, until cheese has melted and sauce is smooth. Serve immediately.

VARIATIONS:

For a different twist, just before serving, stir in 1/4 cup (50 mL) salsa or 1 chopped tomato or 2 cups (500 mL) blanched broccoli florets.

Per adult serving	
CALCIUM	442 mg
VITAMIN D	21 IU
Calories	591
Protein	26 g
Fat	20 g
Carbohydrate	77 g
Dietary Fiber	1 g
Sodium	1096 mg
Magnesium	57 mg

Fettuccine with Mushroom Sauce

Makes 4 servings

The evaporated milk in this sauce is the secret to the heavenly richness. Evaporated milk gives double the calcium while providing the velvety texture of whipping cream but without the fat. For a real treat, use a mixture of white, cremini and portobello mushrooms for an intense mushroom flavor.

1 tbsp	**olive oil**	**15 mL**
1/2 lb	**mushrooms, sliced**	**250 g**
1	**leek, sliced**	**1**
1	**clove garlic, minced**	**1**
1 tbsp	**all-purpose flour**	**15 mL**
1	**can (385 mL) 2% evaporated milk**	**1**
1/2 tsp	**dried thyme**	**2 mL**
1/4 tsp	**pepper**	**1 mL**
1	**pkg (375 g) fettuccine**	**1**
1/4 cup	**chopped fresh parsley**	**50 mL**

1. In saucepan, heat oil over medium heat. Add mushrooms, leek and garlic; cook for 5 minutes or until mushrooms release liquid.
2. Stir in flour; cook, stirring, for 1 minute.
3. Gradually add milk, whisking constantly. Add thyme and pepper; continue to cook, whisking, for 5 minutes or until thickened.
4. In large pot of boiling salted water, cook pasta for 8 to 10 minutes or until al dente. Drain.
5. Toss pasta with mushroom sauce. Garnish with parsley.

Per serving	
CALCIUM	323 mg
VITAMIN D	76 IU
Calories	503
Protein	21 g
Fat	7 g
Carbohydrate	88 g
Dietary Fiber	5 g
Sodium	367 mg
Magnesium	83 mg

Anchovy, Garlic and Broccoli Pasta

This is divine! Even if you hate anchovies, give it a try. This dish has become a Friday-night special at our house because it is fast, easy, a calcium source with anchovies and broccoli, and oh, so tasty. You only need a glass of wine and a salad to think you are in a Mediterranean restaurant.

Makes 3 servings

12 oz	Italian pasta (e.g., orecchiette)	375 g
1	bunch broccoli	1
2 tbsp	extra virgin olive oil	25 mL
1 tbsp	butter	15 mL
1	can (50 g) anchovies, drained and chopped	1
4	cloves garlic, crushed	4
Half	sweet red pepper, chopped	Half
1/4 cup	chopped fresh parsley	50 mL
1 tbsp	lemon juice	15 mL
1/4 tsp	freshly ground black pepper	1 mL
	Freshly grated Parmesan cheese (optional)	

1. In pot of boiling salted water, cook pasta for 8 to 10 minutes, until al dente.
2. Meanwhile, cut broccoli into florets. Discard tough end of stem; peel and thinly slice remaining stem.
3. In large pot of boiling salted water, cook broccoli for 2 to 3 minutes, until tender-crisp; drain. Refresh under cold water.
4. In saucepan, heat oil and butter over medium-high heat. Stir in anchovies and garlic. Add broccoli and red pepper. Stir-fry for 2 minutes. Stir in parsley, lemon juice and pepper.
5. Drain cooked pasta. Toss together pasta and vegetable mixture. Serve immediately with Parmesan cheese (if using).

Per serving	
CALCIUM	136 mg
Calories	617
Protein	23 g
Fat	17 g
Carbohydrate	96 g
Dietary Fiber	9 g
Sodium	826 mg
Magnesium	104 mg

Red and Green Pasta with Almonds

Makes 4 servings

A vibrant pasta with plenty of zing from the calcium vegetables, broccoli and kale, this dish is great served at room temperature.

4 cups	coarsely chopped kale (stems removed)	1 L
2 cups	broccoli florets and sliced peeled stems	500 mL
4 cups	fusilli	1 L
2 tbsp	olive oil	25 mL
2	cloves garlic, minced	2
1 cup	sliced mushrooms	250 mL
1	sweet red pepper, cut in strips	1
2 tbsp	minced fresh tarragon and thyme	25 mL
2 tbsp	balsamic vinegar	25 mL
3/4 tsp	salt	4 mL
1/4 tsp	pepper	1 mL
1/2 cup	toasted whole almonds	125 mL
1/2 cup	chopped green onions	125 mL

1. In large pot of boiling water, cook kale for 5 minutes. Drain in colander; rinse with cold water. Press to remove excess moisture. Set aside.
2. In pot of boiling water, cook broccoli for 3 minutes or until tender-crisp. Rinse under cold water; drain. Add to kale.
3. In large pot of boiling salted water, cook fusilli for 8 to 10 minutes, until al dente.
4. Meanwhile, in large saucepan, heat oil over medium-high heat. Stir in garlic. Add mushrooms; cook, stirring, for 2 minutes.
5. Add red pepper; cook, stirring, for 2 minutes. Add kale and broccoli; cook for 1 minute or until heated through. Remove from heat; stir in herbs, vinegar, salt and pepper.
6. Drain cooked pasta; toss pasta with vegetables. Serve hot or at room temperature, garnished with almonds and green onions.

Per serving	
CALCIUM	148 mg
Calories	522
Protein	17 g
Fat	18 g
Carbohydrate	75 g
Dietary Fiber	8 g
Sodium	677 mg
Magnesium	121 mg

Creamy Red and Green Pasta with Almonds

For added calcium and creaminess, toss the pasta and vegetables in Red and Green Pasta with Almonds (opposite) with this easy sauce.

Makes 4 servings

Red and Green Pasta with Almonds (opposite)

SAUCE:

1 tbsp	olive oil	15 mL
1 tbsp	all-purpose flour	15 mL
1	can (385 mL) 2% evaporated milk	1

1. Sauce: In small saucepan, heat oil over medium-low heat. Whisk in flour; cook, whisking, for 1 minute.
2. Gradually whisk in milk; raise heat to medium. Cook, stirring, for 5 minutes or until thickened.
3. Assembly: Toss sauce with Red and Green Pasta with Almonds. Serve immediately.

Smoked Salmon Linguine

Makes 6 cups (1.5 L) total, 4 servings

Decadent! Rich! Creamy! Evaporated milk gives all the lush, velvety texture and taste of cream but with less fat and all the goodness of extra calcium.

2 tbsp	olive oil	25 mL
3/4 cup	sliced leek (about 1, white and pale green parts only)	175 mL
1	clove garlic, minced	1
1 tbsp	all-purpose flour	15 mL
1	can (385 mL) 2% evaporated milk	1
1	can (7 1/2 oz/213 g) salmon	1
4 oz	smoked salmon, shredded	125 g
1/4 cup	chopped fresh dill	50 mL
2 tbsp	lemon juice	25 mL
1 tsp	grated lemon rind	5 mL
12 oz	linguine	375 g

Evaporated milk has twice the calcium of regular milk and, when thickened with a little flour, acts like whipping cream to create wondrous sauces.

Smoked salmon tidbits work well in this sauce at half the price.

1. In saucepan, heat oil over low heat. Stir in leek and garlic. Lay a piece of waxed paper directly on surface of leek; cover with pot lid. Cook for 10 minutes or until leek is very soft. Remove waxed paper; discard.
2. Increase heat to medium; stir in flour. Cook, stirring, for 1 minute.
3. Gradually whisk in evaporated milk. Cook, stirring, for 5 minutes or until thickened.
4. Drain canned salmon; discard skin. Mash bones; flake salmon. Add to sauce.
5. Add smoked salmon, dill, lemon juice and lemon rind. Cook just until heated through.
6. In large pot of boiling salted water, cook pasta for 8 to 10 minutes, until al dente. Drain.
7. Toss sauce with pasta; serve immediately.

Per serving	
CALCIUM	424 mg
VITAMIN D	285 IU
Calories	579
Protein	33 g
Fat	14 g
Carbohydrate	78 g
Dietary Fiber	4 g
Sodium	736 mg
Magnesium	86 mg

Spaghetti with Turkey Sauce

A lighter version of the usual beef sauce, this turkey version can be served with pasta or rice. Or the sauce can be used in casseroles such as Pasta alla Bolognese (p. 94). To increase calcium, serve with soy pasta and grated Parmesan cheese.

Makes 6 cups/1.5 L sauce, 4 servings

1 lb	soy spaghetti or spaghetti	500 g

TURKEY SAUCE:

1 lb	lean ground turkey or chicken	500 g
3 cups	sliced mushrooms (about 1/2 lb/250 g)	750 mL
2 1/2 cups	chopped onions	625 mL
2	cloves garlic, minced	2
1	can (28 oz/796 mL) diced tomatoes	1
1/4 cup	chopped fresh parsley	50 mL
1/4 cup	tomato paste	50 mL
1 tsp	granulated sugar	5 mL
1 tsp	dried rosemary	5 mL
1	bay leaf	1
	Salt	
	Pepper	

If canned diced tomatoes are unavailable, use canned tomatoes and chop them.

1. Turkey Sauce: In saucepan, cook turkey over medium-high heat for 5 minutes, stirring to break up, until no longer pink. Add mushrooms, onions and garlic; cook, covered, for 5 minutes or until mushrooms and onions are softened.
2. Stir in tomatoes (with juice), parsley, tomato paste, sugar, rosemary and bay leaf. Bring to boil. Reduce heat to medium-low; cook, uncovered, for 20 minutes. Season with salt and pepper to taste.
3. Assembly: Meanwhile, bring separate large pot of salted water to boil. Cook spaghetti for 8 to 10 minutes, until al dente; drain.
4. Remove and discard bay leaf. Serve sauce immediately over spaghetti.

Per 1/2 cup (125 mL) sauce	
CALCIUM	36 mg
Calories	124
Protein	8 g
Fat	7 g
Carbohydrate	8 g
Dietary Fiber	2 g
Sodium	230 mg
Magnesium	23 mg

Per serving	
CALCIUM	142 mg
Calories	797
Protein	41 g
Fat	24 g
Carbohydrate	106 g
Dietary Fiber	10 g
Sodium	972 mg
Magnesium	146 mg

Chapter 8

Casseroles and Vegetables

Many of the calcium-containing vegetables—kale, collards, nappa, bok choy, Chinese cabbage and soybeans—are relatively new to North Americans. If you haven't tried any of these ingredients, you're missing out on some great tastes. Kale and collards are deceptive. They look tough and long-lasting but really should be kept refrigerated and be eaten within a day or two of purchase. Remember to cut away the tough stems.

For convenience, keep a can of soybeans on your shelf. Beans make a great vegetarian meal; use them in hummus, chili or simply as an addition to a salad. A can of baked beans must be the best buy ever! This inexpensive item can make a speedy calcium supper or be transformed into a super tortilla oozing with calcium.

Three-Bean Chili

Makes about 10 cups (2.5 L), 6 servings

Of all the chili recipes I have tried over the years, this one is my favorite. Serve it over rice with a dollop of Drained Yogurt (p. 45) and Tortilla Crisps (p. 53) for a sure way to fight the winter blahs!

2 tbsp	vegetable oil	25 mL
1	large onion, chopped	1
2	cloves garlic, crushed	2
2 tsp	chili powder	10 mL
1 tsp	ground cumin	5 mL
1 tsp	dried oregano	5 mL
1	can (28 oz/796 mL) diced tomatoes	1
3	cans (each 19 oz/540 mL) assorted beans (soy, black and kidney), rinsed and drained	3
1	sweet green pepper, chopped	1
1 tbsp	cider vinegar	15 mL
1/2 tsp	salt	2 mL
1/2 tsp	cinnamon	2 mL
1/4 tsp	pepper	1 mL
1/4 cup	chopped fresh coriander	50 mL

1. In large saucepan, heat oil over medium-high heat. Cook onion and garlic, covered, for 5 minutes or until softened.
2. Stir in chili, cumin and oregano; cook, stirring, for 2 minutes.
3. Stir in tomatoes (with juice). Add beans, green pepper, vinegar, salt, cinnamon and pepper. Bring to boil. Reduce heat to medium-low; simmer for 20 minutes.
4. Just before serving, stir in coriander. Taste for seasoning and adjust if necessary. Chili can be covered and refrigerated for up to 2 days; for longer storage, store in plastic containers and freeze for up to 1 month.

Per serving	
CALCIUM	122 mg
Calories	307
Protein	19 g
Fat	9 g
Carbohydrate	42 g
Dietary Fiber	14 g
Sodium	977 mg
Magnesium	116 mg

VARIATIONS:

For a heartier meal, try turkey, chicken or beef chili—brown 1 lb (500 g) ground turkey, ground chicken or lean ground beef before adding onion and garlic.

A small can of drained corn may be added at the same time as the beans.

Best Beans

This is a relatively quick-cooking method of rehydrating beans from the dry state. Cooking time will vary a little depending on the type of bean used.

Makes 4 cups (1 L)

2 cups	dried navy (pea) beans or soybeans	500 mL
1	whole clove	1
1	onion	1
1	stalk celery	1
1	carrot	1
1	bay leaf	1
2	cloves garlic, cut in half	2
1 tsp	salt	5 mL

1. Rinse beans; put in large pot with 6 cups (1.5 L) water. Bring to boil. Cook at full boil for 10 minutes. Turn heat off. Cover pot; let stand for 1 hour. Drain beans. Return beans to pot.
2. Push clove into onion; add to beans.
3. Add celery, carrot, bay leaf and garlic. Add enough cold water to cover. Bring to boil. Reduce heat to simmer; cook, covered, for 45 minutes. Add salt; simmer for 15 minutes or until beans are tender. Drain beans, discarding vegetables and bay leaf.

Per 1/4 cup (50 mL)	
CALCIUM	41 mg
Calories	83
Protein	5 g
Fat	trace
Carbohydrate	15 g
Dietary Fiber	4 g
Sodium	139 mg
Magnesium	35 mg

Bean Pot

Makes about 2 cups (500 mL), 4 servings

A can of baked beans is a nutrition-packed time-saver. Navy beans (also called pea beans), the basis for baked beans, are a calcium source. Although the method of preparing your own beans (Best Beans, p. 111) has been included in the book, the recipe below can be ready in minutes with a minimum of fuss and maximum taste. You can serve the beans over toast or rice. Or serve the beans with warmed tortillas and accompaniments such as shredded Cheddar, low-fat sour cream, shredded lettuce and chopped chives.

1 tbsp	**vegetable oil**	**15 mL**
1	**large onion, chopped**	**1**
1	**sweet green pepper, coarsely chopped**	**1**
2	**cans (each 14 oz/398 mL) beans in tomato sauce**	**2**
1/4 cup	**salsa**	**50 mL**

1. In saucepan over medium-high heat, heat oil. Cook onion and green pepper, covered, for about 5 minutes or until onion has softened.
2. Stir in beans and salsa.

VARIATION:
To make bean burritos, put a scant 1/2 cup (125 mL) bean mixture at the ends of each of five 10-inch (25 cm) flour tortillas; roll up. Heat in microwave oven or 350°F (180°C) oven until heated through. Serve with bowls of sour cream, salsa, shredded lettuce and shredded Cheddar or Monterey Jack cheese.

Per serving	
CALCIUM	66 mg
Calories	156
Protein	6 g
Fat	4 g
Carbohydrate	28 g
Dietary Fiber	10 g
Sodium	515 mg
Magnesium	41 mg

Anchovy, Garlic and Broccoli Pasta (page 103) with Focaccia (page 98)

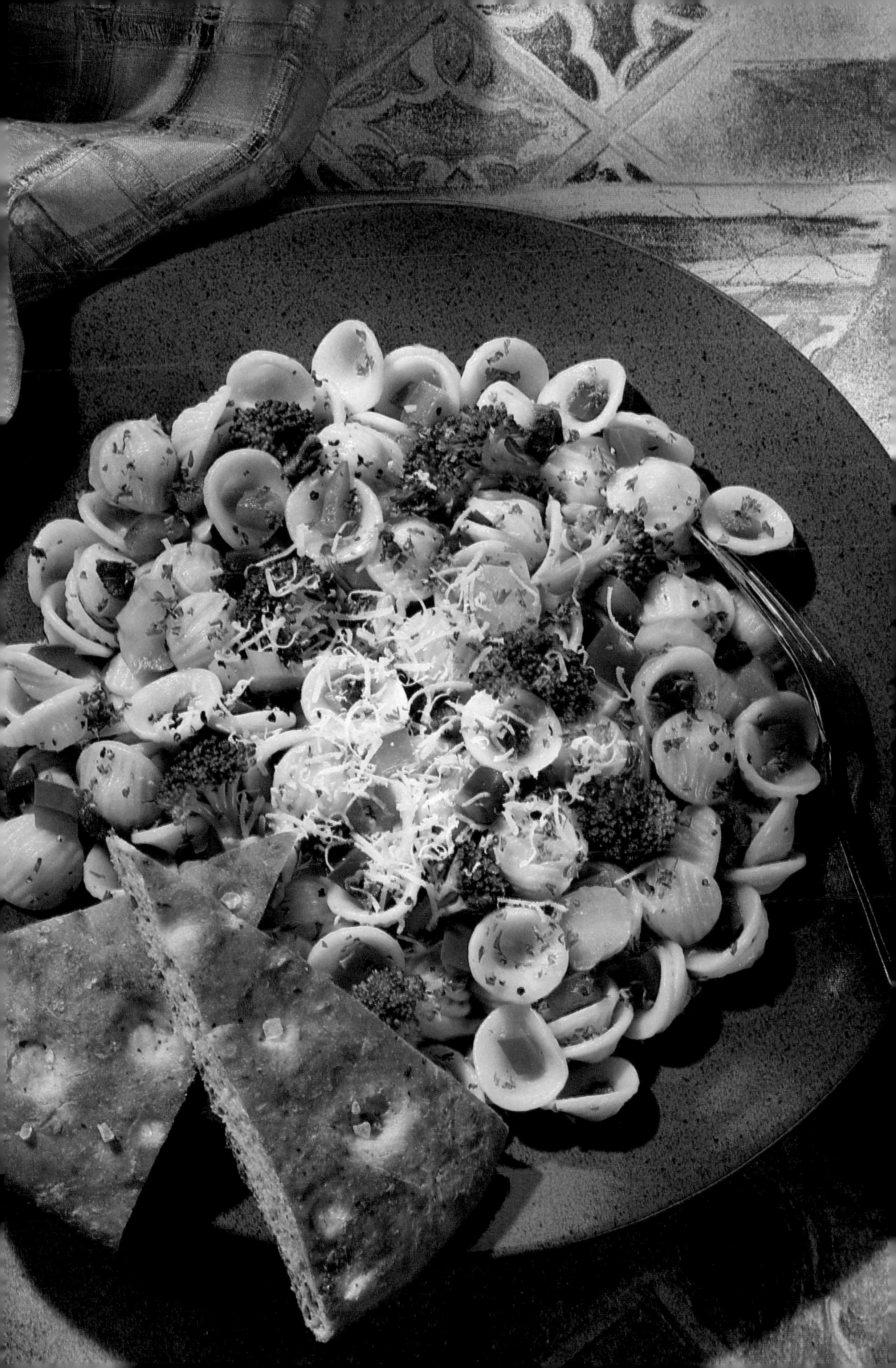

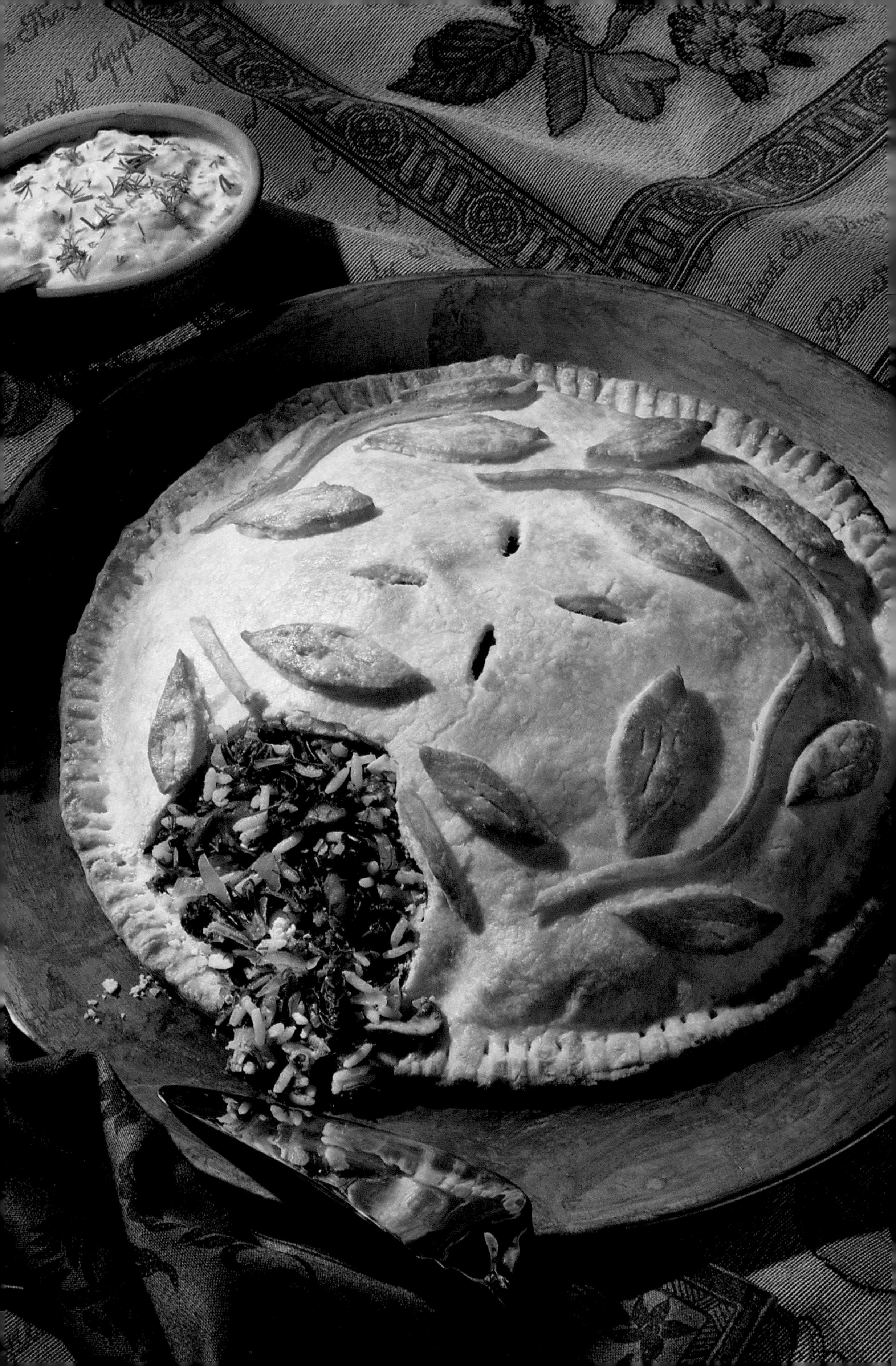

Bok Choy, Nappa and Chinese Cabbage Stir-Fry

If you prepare all your vegetables ahead of time, you can have dinner in minutes. Serve this vegetable combination over a bed of rice or Oriental noodles for a truly authentic-style dinner.

Makes 6 cups (1.5 L), 4 servings

2 tbsp	vegetable oil	25 mL
1	onion, sliced	1
2 tbsp	minced gingerroot	25 mL
2	cloves garlic, minced	2
1/2 tsp	salt	2 mL
3 cups	shredded bok choy	750 mL
3 cups	shredded nappa cabbage	750 mL
3 cups	Chinese cabbage	750 mL
1	sweet red pepper, sliced	1
1/4 cup	chopped fresh coriander	50 mL
1 tbsp	sesame seeds	15 mL
1 tbsp	sesame oil	15 mL
1 tbsp	soy sauce	15 mL

1. In large pot or wok, heat oil over medium-high heat. Add onion, ginger, garlic and salt; stir-fry for 2 minutes. Add bok choy, nappa, Chinese cabbage and red pepper; stir-fry for 3 minutes or until greens are wilted. Remove from heat.
2. Stir in coriander, sesame seeds, sesame oil and soy sauce. Serve immediately.

VARIATIONS:

To turn this into a complete meal, stir in 1 container (10 1/2 oz/297 g) firm tofu, drained and chopped, along with the vegetables.

Or, add 2 cups (500 mL) shredded cooked pork or chicken for a more substantial dish.

Per serving	
CALCIUM	167 mg
Calories	154
Protein	4 g
Fat	12 g
Carbohydrate	10 g
Dietary Fiber	4 g
Sodium	541 mg
Magnesium	38 mg

Kulebiaka of Vegetables and Mushrooms (page 124) with Cucumber-Dill Sauce (page 44)

Broccoli-Feta Soufflé

Makes 6 servings

Eggs are easier to separate when cold, straight from the refrigerator. However, separated egg whites that are at room temperature will whip to a greater volume than cold egg whites.

Even a speck of yolk will prevent the whites from whipping to maximum volume. To ensure yolk-free whites, use three bowls when separating eggs: one to separate eggs over; one to transfer the uncontaminated whites into; and one for the yolks.

Per serving	
CALCIUM	195 mg
VITAMIN D	55 IU
Calories	218
Protein	13 g
Fat	14 g
Carbohydrate	10 g
Dietary Fiber	2 g
Sodium	332 mg
Magnesium	30 mg

Soufflés have a sophisticated reputation, but they are simple in origin—they're basically a cream sauce in which eggs are folded. Soufflés are easy to make, beautiful to behold and heavenly to eat! Serve this nutritious version (with calcium from broccoli, milk and feta) for brunch or an evening meal along with good bread and a salad.

6 cups	broccoli florets and sliced peeled stems (about 1 bunch)	1.5 L
2 tbsp	butter	25 mL
2	cloves garlic, minced	2
1/4 cup	all-purpose flour	50 mL
1 cup	milk or lactose-reduced milk	250 mL
2 tbsp	chopped fresh dill	25 mL
1/4 tsp	pepper	1 mL
Pinch	nutmeg	Pinch
3/4 cup	crumbled feta cheese (about 4 oz/125 g)	175 mL
7	eggs, separated	7
Pinch	salt	Pinch
1 tbsp	freshly grated Parmesan cheese	15 mL

1. Preheat oven to 400°F (200°C). Spray 10-cup (2.5 L) soufflé dish or casserole with nonstick cooking spray.
2. In large pot of boiling water, cook broccoli for 3 minutes or until tender-crisp. Rinse under cold water; drain.
3. In saucepan, melt butter over medium heat. Add garlic; cook for 1 minute, stirring. Add flour; cook, stirring, for 1 minute. Gradually whisk in milk, dill, pepper and nutmeg. (Sauce will be very thick.) Remove from heat.

4. Stir cheese into sauce. Beat 6 of the egg yolks into sauce. Stir in drained broccoli.
5. In large bowl, beat 7 egg whites with salt until soft peaks form. Add one-quarter of the egg whites to broccoli-cheese sauce; fold together. Add remaining egg whites, folding gently. Pour into prepared pan. Sprinkle with Parmesan.
6. Bake in 400°F (200°C) oven for 40 minutes or until puffed and deep brown on top. Serve immediately.

Leftover egg yolks can be used in custards, French toast, scrambled eggs and rice puddings. Keep them covered and refrigerated for up to 2 days.

VARIATION:

You can substitute 8 cups (2 L) chopped stemmed kale (about 1 bunch) for the broccoli. Cook the kale in boiling water for 5 minutes. Rinse under cold water; press out excess moisture. Proceed with recipe.

Kale Balsamic Vinegar Stir-Fry

Makes 2 servings

If you enjoy spinach, you will love this dish. As with spinach, kale wilts to a fraction of its original size once cooked. One large bunch will just serve two people.

8 cups	coarsely chopped kale (stems removed)	2 L
1 tbsp	olive oil	15 mL
1	clove garlic, minced	1
1 tbsp	balsamic vinegar	15 mL

1. In large pot of boiling water, cook kale for 5 minutes. Drain in colander. Rinse with cold water; press to remove excess moisture.
2. In saucepan, heat oil over medium-high heat. Add garlic; stir-fry for 1 minute. Add kale and 1 tbsp (15 mL) water; cook, covered, for 2 minutes.
3. Remove from heat; stir in vinegar. Serve immediately.

Put leftovers on top of grilled bread; sprinkle with shaved Parmesan cheese. Heat under the broiler for kale bruschetta.

Fresh kale does not keep long; use soon after buying. Remove tough center stems from leaves before using. Kale really cooks down: 8 cups (2 L) chopped stemmed kale will yield about 1 cup (250 mL) after blanching.

Per serving	
CALCIUM	206 mg
Calories	154
Protein	5 g
Fat	8 g
Carbohydrate	17 g
Dietary Fiber	6 g
Sodium	65 mg
Magnesium	53 mg

Kale Kannon

Makes 4 servings

An alternative to Colcannon, an Irish mashed potato dish, this recipe is enriched with the calcium from kale.

1 lb	potatoes, peeled and quartered	500 g
4 cups	coarsely chopped kale (stems removed)	1 L
1/2 cup	milk	125 mL
1/4 tsp	salt	1 mL
Pinch	nutmeg	Pinch
Pinch	pepper	Pinch
1 tbsp	chopped green onion or chives	15 mL

1. In saucepan, cover potatoes with cold water. Bring to boil. Reduce heat to medium; cook, covered, for 15 minutes.
2. Add kale to potatoes; cook for 5 minutes. Drain vegetables. Put kale in sieve.
3. Return potatoes to saucepan. Stir in milk, salt, nutmeg and pepper.
4. Using electric mixer, beat potatoes until fluffy and smooth.
5. Press kale to remove excess moisture. Fold kale and green onion into potato mixture. Serve at once.

Per serving	
CALCIUM	97 mg
VITAMIN D	11 IU
Calories	107
Protein	4 g
Fat	1 g
Carbohydrate	22 g
Dietary Fiber	3 g
Sodium	179 mg
Magnesium	34 mg

Kale Soufflé

Makes 6 servings

This soufflé makes a glorious main course or brunch dish. Serve it with salad and crusty bread.

8 cups	coarsely chopped kale (stems removed)	2 L
2 tbsp	butter	25 mL
2	cloves garlic, minced	2
1/4 cup	all-purpose flour	50 mL
1 cup	milk or lactose-reduced milk	250 mL
1/4 tsp	pepper	1 mL
Pinch	nutmeg	Pinch
6	eggs, separated	6
Pinch	salt	Pinch
1 tbsp	freshly grated Parmesan cheese	15 mL

1. Preheat oven to 400°F (200°C). Spray 10-cup (2.5 L) soufflé dish or casserole with nonstick cooking spray.
2. In large pot of boiling water, cook kale for 5 minutes. Drain in colander. Rinse with cold water; press to remove excess moisture.
3. In saucepan, melt butter over medium heat. Add garlic; cook for 1 minute, stirring. Add flour; cook, stirring, for 1 minute. Gradually whisk in milk, pepper and nutmeg. (Sauce will be very thick.) Remove from heat.
4. Beat yolks, one at a time, into sauce. Stir in drained kale.
5. In large bowl, beat egg whites with salt until soft peaks form. Add about one-quarter of the whites to kale sauce; fold together. Add remaining egg whites, folding gently. Pour into prepared pan. Sprinkle with Parmesan.
6. Bake in 400°F (200°C) oven for 40 minutes or until puffed and deep brown on top. Serve immediately.

Per serving

CALCIUM	161 mg
VITAMIN D	49 IU
Calories	181
Protein	10 g
Fat	10 g
Carbohydrate	12 g
Dietary Fiber	2 g
Sodium	164 mg
Magnesium	30 mg

Baked Sweet Potatoes with Almond Pesto Sauce

Makes 4 servings

A baked sweet potato is the ultimate in nutrition, taste and convenience. It is a rich source of beta carotene and, when stuffed with the optional toppings (cheese, sour cream, yogurt or salmon salad), it provides a wallop of calcium. Almond pesto makes a novel topping. Twenty minutes in the microwave oven will produce a satisfying meal for four people.

4	sweet potatoes (about 2 lb/1 kg)	4

ALMOND PESTO SAUCE:

1 cup	coarsely chopped fresh parsley	250 mL
1/4 cup	freshly grated Parmesan cheese	50 mL
2 tbsp	unblanched almonds	25 mL
1 tbsp	dried basil	15 mL
2	cloves garlic, crushed	2
1/2 tsp	salt	2 mL
Pinch	black pepper	Pinch
1/3 cup	extra virgin olive oil	75 mL

1. Scrub sweet potatoes; using fork, prick potatoes in several places. Microwave at High for 20 minutes. Let stand for 2 minutes.
2. Almond Pesto Sauce: Meanwhile, in food processor, combine parsley, cheese, almonds, basil, garlic, salt and pepper; process until finely chopped. With motor running, pour oil through feed tube. Purée until smooth.
3. Assembly: Make a slit in each potato; squeeze potato open. Place 1 tbsp (15 mL) of almond pesto in each slit. Serve at once. Any leftover pesto can be frozen to serve later with pasta or spread on pizza.

Per serving	
CALCIUM	90 mg
Calories	242
Protein	4 g
Fat	8 g
Carbohydrate	41 g
Dietary Fiber	5 g
Sodium	160 mg
Magnesium	41 mg

Vegetable Soufflé

Makes 4 servings

Serve this as a vegetarian main course with a salad, such as the Oriental Coleslaw (p. 82), and Whole Wheat Calcium-Yeast Bread (p. 30). Of course, this soufflé would make an ideal companion to a turkey or roast pork dinner, too! Not as fragile as some of its cousins, this soufflé, although best served hot, can stand for about 20 minutes before serving, making it ideal for a buffet.

Eggs are easier to separate when cold, straight from the refrigerator. However, separated egg whites that are at room temperature will whip to a greater volume than cold egg whites.

Even a speck of yolk will prevent the whites from whipping to maximum volume. To ensure yolk-free whites, use three bowls when separating eggs: one to separate eggs over; one to transfer the uncontaminated whites into; and one for the yolks.

2 cups	puréed cooked carrot, parsnip, rutabaga, squash or sweet potato	500 mL
2	eggs, separated	2
1 cup	shredded old Cheddar cheese	250 mL
1/4 cup	instant skim milk powder	50 mL
1/4 tsp	salt	1 mL
Pinch	nutmeg	Pinch
Pinch	salt	Pinch

1. Preheat oven to 375°F (190°C). Spray a 4- to 6-cup (1 to 1.5 L) soufflé or gratin dish with nonstick cooking spray.
2. In bowl, beat together puréed vegetable, egg yolks, cheese, skim milk powder, the 1/4 tsp (1 mL) salt and nutmeg.
3. In separate bowl, beat egg whites with the pinch of salt until soft peaks form.
4. Add about one-quarter of the whites to vegetable mixture; fold together. Gently fold in remaining whites.
5. Pour mixture into prepared dish; smooth out top. Bake in 375°F (190°C) oven for 35 to 40 minutes or until browned on top. Serve hot.

Per serving	
CALCIUM	304 mg
VITAMIN D	36 IU
Calories	217
Protein	13 g
Fat	12 g
Carbohydrate	15 g
Dietary Fiber	3 g
Sodium	448 mg
Magnesium	30 mg

Chapter 9

Main Courses

Soy, in the form of tofu, is the main event. It is a great calcium-containing protein food for vegetarians. Soy also combines well with other ingredients. Likewise, canned salmon offers versatility, too: use it in dips, salads or as a stunning calcium-enriched kulebiaka recipe. In this chapter, you will find a wide variety of recipes in which protein foods are deliciously combined with calcium-containing vegetables, almonds and sesame seeds.

Savory Salmon Cakes

Makes four 2-inch (5 cm) patties or two 3-inch (7.5 cm) patties

Serve these savory treats on a sesame bun with cucumber slices for a quick-and-easy meal with a calcium punch! For more upscale party fare, serve appetizer-size patties with a refreshing Cucumber-Dill Sauce (p. 44) for dipping.

COATING:

1 cup	**fresh bread crumbs (preferably whole wheat)**	**250 mL**
1/4 cup	**toasted chopped almonds**	**50 mL**
1/4 cup	**sesame seeds**	**50 mL**
1 tbsp	**dried tarragon**	**15 mL**
1/2 tsp	**salt**	**2 mL**

PATTIES:

1	**can (7 1/2 oz/213 g) salmon**	**1**
1/2 cup	**fresh bread crumbs (preferably whole wheat)**	**125 mL**
1	**egg**	**1**
1 tbsp	**light salad dressing**	**15 mL**
1 tbsp	**1% plain yogurt**	**15 mL**
1/2 tsp	**dried tarragon**	**2 mL**
1/4 tsp	**pepper**	**1 mL**

1. Coating: In bowl, combine bread crumbs, almonds, sesame seeds, tarragon and salt.
2. Patties: Drain salmon; remove and discard skin. In separate bowl, combine salmon (including bones), bread crumbs, egg, salad dressing, yogurt, tarragon and pepper; mix well.

Per 3-inch (7.5 cm) patty	
CALCIUM	340 mg
VITAMIN D	436 IU
Calories	372
Protein	28 g
Fat	20 g
Carbohydrate	23 g
Dietary Fiber	4 g
Sodium	1199 mg
Magnesium	82 mg

3. Assembly: Divide salmon mixture into 2 or 4 equal portions; form into patties. Coat with bread-crumb coating.
4. Spray nonstick frying pan with nonstick cooking spray. Preheat pan over medium-high heat. Add patties; immediately reduce heat to medium. Cook for about 5 minutes per side or until golden brown and heated through.

Pie Pastry

A good basic recipe, this pastry is enriched with calcium by the addition of soy flour. Use it with sweet or savory fillings. Because this pastry is made with shortening rather than butter, it is suitable for those with lactose intolerance.

Makes pastry for one 9-inch (23 cm) double-crust pie or two 9-inch (23 cm) single-crust pies

1 1/2 cups	**all-purpose flour**	**375 mL**
1/2 cup	**soy flour**	**125 mL**
1/2 tsp	**salt**	**2 mL**
3/4 cup	**shortening**	**175 mL**
1/3 cup	**cold water**	**75 mL**

1. In mixing bowl, stir together all-purpose flour, soy flour and salt. Using pastry cutter or 2 knives, cut shortening into flour mixture until mixture resembles fine crumbs. Stir in water. Divide mixture in half; form each half into ball. Between 2 sheets of waxed paper, roll each ball to fit 9-inch (23 cm) pie plate.

Per 1/8 double crust

CALCIUM	15 mg
Calories	270
Protein	5 g
Fat	19 g
Carbohydrate	20 g
Dietary Fiber	1 g
Sodium	145 mg
Magnesium	22 mg

Kulebiaka of Vegetables and Mushrooms

Makes 8 servings

This main course of Russian origin is fantastic for a buffet. It looks and tastes divine. You can make it ahead and freeze for frazzle-free entertaining AND the ingredients won't break the bank! For maximum flavor, splurge on portobello or cremini mushrooms if they're available; otherwise, use the common white mushroom. This dish would go well with the Cucumber-Dill Sauce (p. 44).

FILLING:

1/4 cup	wild rice	50 mL
1	bay leaf	1
3/4 cup	water	175 mL
1 cup	vegetable stock	250 mL
1/2 cup	parboiled long-grain or brown rice	125 mL
4 cups	coarsely chopped kale (stems removed)	1 L
2 tbsp	extra virgin olive oil	25 mL
4 cups	sliced cabbage (red or green)	1 L
2 cups	sliced mushrooms	500 mL
1	large onion, chopped	1
1/2 cup	chopped fresh parsley	125 mL
1/2 cup	crumbled drained firm tofu or 2 chopped hard-cooked eggs	125 mL
1/4 cup	chopped fresh dill	50 mL
1/4 cup	lemon juice	50 mL
1/2 tsp	salt	2 mL
1/4 tsp	freshly ground black pepper	1 mL

NO-FUSS YOGURT PUFF PASTRY:

2 cups	all-purpose flour	500 mL
1 tsp	baking powder	5 mL
1/2 tsp	salt	2 mL
1/2 cup	butter	125 mL
1/4 cup	shortening	50 mL
1/2 cup	1% plain yogurt	125 mL

Per serving	
CALCIUM	136 mg
VITAMIN D	5 IU
Calories	431
Protein	10 g
Fat	24 g
Carbohydrate	46 g
Dietary Fiber	4 g
Sodium	552 mg
Magnesium	47 mg

EGG WASH:

1	egg	1
1 tbsp	milk or water	15 mL

1. Preheat oven to 425°F (220°C). Spray baking sheet with nonstick cooking spray.
2. Filling: In small bowl, soak wild rice in enough cold water to cover for 30 minutes. Drain. In small saucepan, bring bay leaf and the 3/4 cup (175 mL) water to boil. Stir in wild rice. Reduce heat to medium-low. Cook, covered, for 15 minutes. Remove from heat; let stand for 5 minutes. Discard bay leaf.
3. Meanwhile, in small saucepan, bring stock to boil. Stir in long-grain rice. Reduce heat to medium-low. Cook, covered, for 15 minutes. Remove from heat; let stand for 5 minutes.
4. Meanwhile, in large pot of boiling water, cook kale for 5 minutes. Drain in colander. Rinse with cold water, pressing to remove excess moisture.
5. In saucepan, heat oil over medium-high heat. Add cabbage, mushrooms and onion; cook, covered, for 5 minutes or until tender.
6. In large bowl, combine wild rice, long-grain rice, kale, cabbage mixture, parsley, tofu, dill, lemon juice, salt and pepper.
7. No-Fuss Yogurt Puff Pastry: In bowl, stir together flour, baking powder and salt.
8. Using pastry blender or two knives, cut butter and shortening into flour mixture until mixture resembles fine crumbs. Using fork, stir in yogurt; form dough into ball.

To bake "blind" (that is, baking pastry without a filling) prick the base of the pastry with a fork; line the pastry shell with parchment paper and sprinkle with about 3 cups (750 mL) rice or dried beans. Bake in 425°F (220°C) oven for about 20 minutes. Carefully remove rice or beans (save in a jar for another time) and parchment paper. Return pastry shell to oven and continue baking for about 10 minutes or until golden brown.

Although soy flour is available in two forms, high fat and low fat, the recipes were tested using low fat. You can use either.

Always use shortening at room temperature; it makes working it into the flour mixture much easier.

9. Divide dough into two portions: 2/3 and 1/3. Roll out the 1/3 portion between 2 sheets of waxed paper to make 10-inch (25 cm) circle. Gently remove top sheet of waxed paper; invert pastry onto prepared baking sheet. Between waxed paper, roll the 2/3 dough portion to 12 inches (30 cm).
10. Assembly: Press vegetable filling into mound on pastry base. Invert larger pastry sheet over filling, gently shaping over filling, trimming and crimping edges to make neat circle. Set aside pastry trimmings.
11. Egg Wash: In small bowl, whisk together egg and milk. Brush over pastry surface.
12. Assembly: Between 2 sheets of waxed paper, roll pastry trimmings to 1/4-inch (5 mm) thickness. Using sharp knife or small cookie cutter, cut out shapes. Lay pastry shapes on top of pie in decorative pattern. Cut vents into pastry.
13. Bake in 425°F (220°C) oven for 25 to 35 minutes or until golden brown. Serve hot or at room temperature. Recipe may be made 1 day ahead and stored in refrigerator. For longer storage, wrap well and freeze for up to 1 month.

VARIATIONS:

Instead of using a baking sheet, use a 9-inch (23 cm) pie plate.

Use Pie Pastry (p. 123) instead of the puff pastry if lactose-intolerant.

Instead of this filling, try the Salmon-Rice Casserole (p. 96) as the filling for a change of pace.

If you prefer, delete the pastry and serve the filling as a vegetable casserole.

Crispy Oven-Baked Chicken

A calcium-enriched, crunchy coating on this skinless chicken keeps it moist and tender inside, while cutting down on the fat at the same time. Serve hot or cold with a colorful garden salad and creamy mashed potatoes for a nutritious comfort meal.

Makes 8 servings

2 cups	fresh bread crumbs (preferably whole wheat)	500 mL
1/2 cup	toasted chopped almonds	125 mL
1/4 cup	sesame seeds	50 mL
1 tbsp	dried tarragon	15 mL
1/2 tsp	salt	2 mL
1/2 cup	1% plain yogurt	125 mL
2 tbsp	light salad dressing	25 mL
1 tbsp	Dijon mustard	15 mL
4 to 5 lb	chicken legs (8) or breasts (10)	2 to 2.5 kg

1. Preheat oven to 350°F (180°C). Spray 13- x 9-inch (3.5 L) baking dish with nonstick cooking spray.
2. In bowl, combine bread crumbs, almonds, sesame seeds, tarragon and salt.
3. In separate bowl, combine yogurt, salad dressing and mustard.
4. Remove skin and all visible fat from chicken pieces. Coat generously with yogurt mixture.
5. Transfer bread-crumb mixture to plate or shallow pan. Dip chicken pieces into crumbs, coating both sides. Arrange chicken in prepared baking dish.
6. Bake in 350°F (180°C) oven for about 1 1/4 hours or until juices run clear when chicken is pierced with fork and coating is golden.

VARIATION:
For a lactose-free variation, substitute light salad dressing for the yogurt.

Any leftover coating that has been in contact with raw chicken should be discarded for food safety.

Cooked chicken will keep refrigerated for up to 2 days.

Per serving	
CALCIUM	82 mg
Calories	281
Protein	31 g
Fat	13 g
Carbohydrate	10 g
Dietary Fiber	2 g
Sodium	357 mg
Magnesium	67 mg

Broccoli-Mushroom Pie

Makes 8 servings

A substantial vegetarian pie that reheats well, this dish's festive appearance and flavor marry well with chutney, whole wheat bread and a green salad.

WHOLE WHEAT SESAME SEED PASTRY:

3/4 cup	whole wheat flour	175 mL
3/4 cup	all-purpose flour	175 mL
1/2 cup	soy flour	125 mL
1/2 tsp	salt	2 mL
3/4 cup	shortening (at room temperature)	175 mL
2 tbsp	sesame seeds	25 mL
1/3 cup	cold water	75 mL

BROCCOLI-MUSHROOM FILLING:

1	bunch broccoli (2 stalks)	1
2 tbsp	olive oil	25 mL
8 oz	mushrooms, sliced	250 g
1	onion, chopped	1
1 cup	diced sweet red pepper	250 mL
2	cloves garlic, minced	2
1 tsp	dried oregano	5 mL
1/2 tsp	dried thyme	2 mL
1/2 tsp	salt	2 mL
1/4 tsp	black pepper	1 mL
8 oz	silken tofu (or 4 oz/125 g cream cheese)	250 g
1 cup	fresh brown bread crumbs	250 mL
1/2 cup	milk or soy beverage	125 mL
1/4 cup	freshly grated Parmesan cheese	50 mL
1/4 cup	minced fresh parsley	50 mL
2 tbsp	lemon juice	25 mL
2	eggs, beaten	2

1. Preheat oven to 425°F (220°C). Whole Wheat Sesame Seed Pastry: In mixing bowl or food processor using steel blade, combine whole wheat flour, all-purpose flour, soy flour and salt.

Per serving	
CALCIUM	125 mg
VITAMIN D	9 IU
Calories	391
Protein	13 g
Fat	26 g
Carbohydrate	30 g
Dietary Fiber	5 g
Sodium	414 mg
Magnesium	58 mg

2. Cut shortening into cubes; add to flour mixture. Using pastry cutter or steel blade of food processor, cut shortening into flour mixture until mixture resembles fine crumbs. Stir in sesame seeds.
3. Pour water over flour mixture; combine just until dough sticks together.
4. Remove dough from bowl; form into ball.
5. Divide dough in half. Roll 1 half between 2 sheets of waxed paper. Gripping paper firmly between tummy and counter edge, roll dough away from you to form circle about 12 inches (30 cm) in diameter. Repeat with remaining dough.
6. Carefully lift waxed paper from pastry; invert 1 pastry circle into 9-inch (23 cm) pie plate. Set aside other pastry circle for top crust. Cut top layer into lattice.
7. Filling: Cut broccoli into florets. Peel and thinly slice stems. Steam broccoli until tender-crisp. Set aside.
8. In large saucepan, over medium-high heat, heat oil. Sauté mushrooms, onion, red pepper, garlic, oregano, thyme, salt and pepper until onions are soft.
9. In bowl, crumble tofu; stir in broccoli, bread crumbs, milk, Parmesan, parsley and lemon juice. Stir in all but 1 tbsp (15 mL) of the eggs. Combine well.
10. Assembly: Spoon filling into prepared pie shell; cover with pastry lattice. Mix reserved egg with 1 tbsp (15 mL) water; brush over pastry.
11. Bake in 425°F (220°C) oven for 15 minutes. Reduce heat to 350°F (180°C) and bake for 30 to 40 minutes or until pastry is deep golden. Let cool for at least 20 minutes before serving. For best flavor, make 1 day ahead and reheat at 350°F (180°C) for about 20 minutes.

Sweet Potato Shepherd's Pie

Makes 4 servings

This old-timer gets a new face with a sweet potato topping and turkey filling. Both the milk and skim milk powder whipped into the potatoes will give readily absorbed calcium. Likewise, the turkey filling has been enriched with skim milk powder and evaporated milk—simple ways in which many popular recipes can be enriched with calcium.

TOPPING:

2 1/2 lb	sweet potatoes, peeled and quartered	1.25 kg
1/2 cup	instant skim milk powder (optional)	125 mL
1/2 cup	milk or soy beverage	125 mL
1/2 tsp	salt	2 mL
1/4 tsp	pepper	1 mL

BASE:

1 lb	lean ground turkey	500 g
3 cups	sliced mushrooms (about 8 oz/ 250 g)	750 mL
1 cup	chopped onion	250 mL
1/2 cup	chopped celery	125 mL
2	cloves garlic, minced	2
1/2 tsp	salt	2 mL
1/4 tsp	pepper	1 mL
1/4 tsp	dried thyme	1 mL
2 tbsp	instant skim milk powder	25 mL
2 tbsp	minced fresh parsley	25 mL
1 tbsp	all-purpose flour	15 mL
1/2 cup	2% evaporated milk or soy beverage	125 mL

Per serving	
CALCIUM	255 mg
VITAMIN D	44 IU
Calories	560
Protein	30 g
Fat	21 g
Carbohydrate	64 g
Dietary Fiber	8 g
Sodium	732 mg
Magnesium	88 mg

1. Preheat oven to 350°F (180°C). Spray 8-cup (2 L) baking dish with nonstick cooking spray.
2. Topping: In saucepan, cover sweet potatoes with cold water. Bring to boil. Reduce heat to medium; cook, covered, for 12 to 15 minutes or until tender when pierced with tip of knife. Drain; mash potatoes with skim milk powder (if using), milk, salt and pepper.
3. Base: In large saucepan, cook turkey over medium-high heat for 5 to 7 minutes, stirring to break up, until no longer pink. Add mushrooms, onion, celery, garlic, salt, pepper and thyme. Cook, covered, for 10 minutes.
4. Stir in skim milk powder, parsley and flour. Gradually stir in evaporated milk.
5. Assembly: Transfer turkey mixture to prepared baking dish. Spoon or pipe potato topping onto turkey mixture. Bake in 350°F (180°C) oven for 40 to 45 minutes, until heated through.

Tofu Tourtière

Makes 6 servings

For years, tourtière has been a traditional Christmas pie served for the festivities and also during the winter months. Tofu Tourtière is an updated version appealing to vegetarians and those who prefer lighter fare. Serve this with Cranberry-Orange Chutney (p. 43) for a seasonal treat.

Soy flour is available in two forms: high fat and low fat. Low fat was used in developing the recipes, but either will work.

Use flat-leaf Italian parsley for extra flavor.

PASTRY:

1 1/2 cups	all-purpose flour	375 mL
1/2 cup	soy flour	125 mL
1/2 tsp	salt	2 mL
3/4 cup	shortening	175 mL
1/3 cup	cold water	75 mL

FILLING:

3 cups	fresh bread crumbs (preferably whole wheat)	750 mL
2 tbsp	vegetable oil	25 mL
12 oz	mushrooms, chopped	375 g
2 cups	sliced leeks	500 mL
1	clove garlic, minced	1
1 tsp	dried thyme	5 mL
1 tsp	salt	5 mL
1/2 tsp	nutmeg	2 mL
1/2 tsp	pepper	2 mL
8 oz	firm tofu, crumbled	250 g
1 1/2 cups	vegetable stock	375 mL
1/4 cup	minced fresh parsley	50 mL
1	egg, beaten	1

1. Preheat oven to 350°F (180°C).
2. Pastry: In mixing bowl, stir together all-purpose flour, soy flour and salt. Using pastry cutter or two knives, cut shortening into flour mixture until mixture resembles fine crumbs. Stir in water. Divide mixture in half; form each half into ball. Between 2 sheets of waxed paper, roll each

Per serving	
CALCIUM	142 mg
VITAMIN D	6 IU
Calories	540
Protein	17 g
Fat	35 g
Carbohydrate	44 g
Dietary Fiber	6 g
Sodium	914 mg
Magnesium	76 mg

ball to fit 9-inch (23 cm) pie plate. Line bottom of 9-inch (23 cm) pie plate with pastry; refrigerate pie plate and top crust.

3. Filling: Spread bread crumbs on baking sheet; bake in 350°F (180°C) oven for 15 minutes or until golden. Increase oven temperature to 450°F (230°C).
4. In large saucepan, heat oil over medium heat. Cook mushrooms, leeks, garlic, thyme, salt, nutmeg and pepper for 5 minutes or until mushrooms give up their juices. Remove from heat. Stir in bread crumbs, tofu, vegetable stock and parsley. Let cool to room temperature. Taste for seasoning; adjust if necessary. Stir in egg.
5. Assembly: Spoon filling into prepared pastry shell. Cover with top crust. Flute edges; using sharp knife, slash steam vents into top crust.
6. Bake in 450°F (230°C) oven for 10 minutes. Reduce heat to 375°F (190°C); bake for 30 minutes or until golden brown. Let stand for 15 minutes. Cut into wedges and serve immediately or serve at room temperature. For best flavor, make tourtière 1 day ahead and store it in refrigerator; reheat in 350°F (180°C) oven for 20 to 25 minutes.

VARIATIONS:

For extra mushroomy flavor, use oyster, shiitake or porcini mushrooms for all or part of the mushrooms.

TURKEY TOURTIÈRE

Substitute 1 1/2 lb (750 g) ground turkey or ground chicken for the tofu; decrease the amount of mushrooms to 8 oz (250 g) and the dried thyme to 1/2 tsp (2 mL). Replace the vegetable stock with turkey or chicken stock and omit the egg. Prepare as for Tofu Tourtière.

Chapter 10

Sweet Endings

Drained yogurt, cottage cheese, evaporated milk and ricotta replace the richness of whipping cream and cream cheese in the usual ultra-decadent dessert. There is much less fat with these substitutes, but there is no sacrifice of flavor. Toasted almonds, molasses, dried figs and dried apricots along with the spark of grated orange and orange juice add zest to sweets. To raise the calcium content of baked goods, soy flour is substituted for some of the all-purpose flour, while cookies are dipped into sesame seeds for a final decorative flourish of calcium.

Cake fillings and frostings can have calcium too. Drained yogurt sauce can be served as a sauce for sweets such as cake. Try making the Frozen Lemon Yogurt, but do not freeze it. Instead of using it as a frozen dessert, you can prepare it as a lemon filling for cakes and tartlets. Almonds and ricotta also create delectable calcium fillings that replace the cloying sweetness of their butter-cream cousins. These are just a few of the countless ways to enliven dessert and cookie recipes with calcium.

Almond Shortbread

Makes about 4 dozen

Crispy, buttery and melt-in-your-mouth, these are the ultimate shortbread, with a bonus—added calcium from soy flour and almonds.

2 cups	all-purpose flour	500 mL
1/2 cup	toasted chopped almonds	125 mL
1/4 cup	soy flour or all-purpose flour	50 mL
1 cup	butter, softened	250 mL
2/3 cup	granulated sugar	150 mL
1/2 tsp	almond extract	2 mL

1. Preheat oven to 350°F (180°C). Line baking sheet with parchment paper.
2. In mixing bowl, stir together all-purpose flour, almonds and soy flour.
3. In separate bowl, using electric mixer, beat together butter, sugar and almond extract until fluffy. Gradually beat in flour mixture, 1/2 cup (125 mL) at a time, scraping down sides of bowl occasionally.
4. Between 2 sheets of waxed paper, roll dough out to 1/4-inch (5 mm) thickness. Remove top layer of paper. Using fancy cookie cutter, cut out cookies; arrange cookies on prepared baking sheet. Reroll dough between waxed paper and continue to cut out cookies until all dough is used up.
5. Bake in 350°F (180°C) oven for 20 to 25 minutes or until golden brown. Store shortbread in cookie tin at room temperature for up to 1 week. For longer storage, wrap well and freeze for up to 3 months.

After dough is made, form into ball. Dip ball into flour. Dough will roll more easily and will not stick to waxed paper.

Soy flour is available in two forms: high fat and low fat. This recipe was tested with low-fat soy flour.

If dough becomes sticky and hard to work with, refrigerate it to firm it up.

To toast almonds, place them in a baking dish and bake in 350°F (180°C) oven for 12 to 15 minutes or until golden brown and fragrant.

Per piece	
CALCIUM	7 mg
Calories	73
Protein	1 g
Fat	5 g
Carbohydrate	7 g
Dietary Fiber	trace
Sodium	39 mg
Magnesium	7 mg

Chocolate-Apricot Chews

Who can resist chocolate, especially when it's teamed up with chewy apricots, crunchy toasted almonds and sesame seeds?

Makes 36 squares or 48 truffles

1/2 cup	chopped dried apricots	125 mL
4 cups	quick-cooking rolled oats	1 L
1/2 cup	chopped unblanched almonds, toasted	125 mL
1 cup	sesame seeds, divided	250 mL
1 1/2 cups	granulated sugar	375 mL
1/2 cup	unsweetened cocoa powder	125 mL
1/2 cup	butter	125 mL
1/2 cup	milk	125 mL
1 tbsp	vanilla extract	15 mL

A glass of cold milk is the perfect partner for these no-bake bars, not to mention an excellent source of calcium. As a bonus, the bars can be easily transformed into truffles, too.

1. Line 9-inch (2.5 L) square pan with waxed paper if making squares.
2. In small bowl, pour enough boiling water to cover over apricots; let stand for 1 minute. Drain.
3. In mixing bowl, stir together apricots, oats, almonds and half of the sesame seeds.
4. In large saucepan, whisk together sugar, cocoa, butter, milk and vanilla. Bring mixture to boil; cook over medium-high heat for 2 minutes, whisking frequently.
5. Remove saucepan from heat. Pour oat mixture into cocoa mixture, stirring to combine well.
6. If making squares, when mixture is cool enough to handle, after about 5 minutes, spoon into prepared pan. Sprinkle with remaining sesame seeds; press seeds down. Let cool thoroughly before cutting into squares. (If making truffles, while mixture is still warm, form 1-inch/2.5 cm balls using about 1 tbsp/15 mL batter; roll balls in remaining sesame seeds.) Chews may be kept covered and refrigerated for up to 1 week. For longer storage, wrap well and freeze for up to 3 months.

Per square	
CALCIUM	23 mg
VITAMIN D	1 IU
Calories	136
Protein	3 g
Fat	7 g
Carbohydrate	17 g
Dietary Fiber	2 g
Sodium	40 mg
Magnesium	35 mg

Molasses Crinkles

Makes 48 crinkles

An old-fashioned recipe with a new calcium face, these crinkles are enriched with molasses, soy flour and sesame seeds.

3/4 cup	shortening	175 mL
3/4 cup	granulated sugar	175 mL
1	egg	1
1/4 cup	molasses	50 mL
1 1/2 cups	cake-and-pastry flour	375 mL
1/2 cup	soy flour	125 mL
2 tsp	baking soda	10 mL
1 tsp	cinnamon	5 mL
1 tsp	ground ginger	5 mL
1 tsp	ground cloves	5 mL
1/3 cup	sesame seeds	75 mL

Blackstrap molasses contain more calcium than 'table' or 'fancy' molasses.

1. Preheat oven to 350°F (180°C). Grease baking sheet or spray with nonstick cooking spray.
2. In mixing bowl, using electric mixer, beat shortening and sugar together until creamy. Beat in egg until fluffy. Stir in molasses.
3. In separate bowl, sift together cake-and-pastry flour, soy flour, baking soda, cinnamon, ginger and cloves.
4. Gradually beat flour mixture into creamed mixture until well combined.
5. Roll dough into about 48 balls (about 1 tbsp/15 mL each). Roll each ball in sesame seeds.
6. Arrange on prepared baking sheet. Bake in 350°F (180°C) oven for 10 to 12 minutes or until slightly flattened. Let cool for 10 minutes before removing to rack. Crinkles may be stored in cookie tin at room temperature for up to 1 week. For longer storage, wrap well and freeze for up to 3 months.

Per cookie	
CALCIUM	9 mg
Calories	70
Protein	1 g
Fat	4 g
Carbohydrate	7 g
Dietary Fiber	trace
Sodium	51 mg
Magnesium	10 mg

Fruited Truffles

I consider these a self-righteous version. Calcium-enhanced, bursting with flavor and low in fat, these truffles are the answer to decadence for the health-conscious.

Makes about 30 truffles

1 cup	chopped dried figs	250 mL
1 cup	chopped dates	250 mL
1 cup	toasted chopped almonds	250 mL
2 tbsp	lemon juice	25 mL
1 tbsp	grated orange rind	15 mL
1 tbsp	grated lemon rind	15 mL
2 tbsp	granulated sugar	25 mL
2 tbsp	sesame seeds	25 mL

1. In food processor, combine figs, dates and almonds until finely chopped.
2. Add lemon juice, orange rind and lemon rind; process until well combined.
3. In small bowl, combine sugar and sesame seeds.
4. Roll 1 tbsp (15 mL) fruit mixture into ball; then roll in sugar-sesame mixture. Repeat to make 30 truffles. Store fruit truffles in container in refrigerator for up to 1 week. For longer storage, wrap well and freeze for up to 3 months.

Per truffle	
CALCIUM	24 mg
Calories	66
Protein	1 g
Fat	3 g
Carbohydrate	10 g
Dietary Fiber	1 g
Sodium	2 mg
Magnesium	22 mg

Spectacular Spicy Biscotti

Makes about 36 pieces

Sample this new twist on biscotti. It has Middle Eastern overtones with the dried figs which provide extra calcium goodness. For fun, substitute dates or apricots for the figs. Both the flavor and the calcium content get a boost from the soy flour, almonds, sesame seeds and molasses.

1 1/2 cups	all-purpose flour	375 mL
1 cup	chopped dried figs	250 mL
1/2 cup	soy flour or all-purpose flour	125 mL
1/2 cup	packed brown sugar	125 mL
1/2 cup	toasted chopped almonds	125 mL
1 1/2 tsp	cinnamon	7 mL
1 tsp	baking powder	5 mL
1/2 tsp	baking soda	2 mL
1/2 tsp	ground cardamom	2 mL
1/2 tsp	ground ginger	2 mL
1/2 tsp	salt	2 mL
2	eggs	2
1/3 cup	molasses	75 mL
1 tbsp	grated lemon rind	15 mL
1/4 cup	sesame seeds	50 mL

1. Preheat oven to 325°F (160°C). Line baking sheet with parchment paper.
2. In bowl, combine all-purpose flour, figs, soy flour, brown sugar, almonds, cinnamon, baking powder, baking soda, cardamom, ginger and salt.
3. In separate bowl, whisk together eggs, molasses and lemon rind.
4. Stir egg mixture into flour mixture until well mixed. Dough will be stiff.

Per piece	
CALCIUM	30 mg
VITAMIN D	2 IU
Calories	76
Protein	2 g
Fat	2 g
Carbohydrate	13 g
Dietary Fiber	1 g
Sodium	62 mg
Magnesium	19 mg

5. Divide dough into 2 equal portions. Shape each into log 6 x 2 x 1 inch (15 x 5 x 2.5 cm). Roll logs in sesame seeds to cover. Place on prepared baking sheet.
6. Bake in 325°F (160°C) oven for 40 to 50 minutes, until pale brown. Let cool on racks.
7. Using sharp knife, slice logs on the diagonal at 1/2-inch (1 cm) intervals. Arrange slices on same baking sheet.
8. Bake in 350°F (180°C) oven for 10 minutes. Let cool on racks. Store in cookie tins at room temperature for up to 1 week. For longer storage, wrap well and freeze for up to 2 months.

Marzipan Truffles

These delicate morsels are a welcome addition on a sweet tray or in a candy box.

Makes 18 truffles

	Marzipan (p. 46 or use (8 oz/500 g) store-bought)	
18	**whole unblanched almonds**	18

1. Divide marzipan into 18 pieces (each about 2 tsp/10 mL); roll each into ball.
2. Press an almond into center of each marzipan ball. Place on plate; cover and refrigerate for at least 1 hour before serving. Keeps refrigerated for 1 week. For longer storage, wrap well and freeze for up to 3 months.

Per truffle	
CALCIUM	16 mg
Calories	61
Protein	1 g
Fat	3 g
Carbohydrate	7 g
Dietary Fiber	trace
Sodium	4 mg
Magnesium	18 mg

Orange Liqueur Biscotti

Makes about 30 pieces

A cup of coffee and a biscotti make ideal partners. Biscotti are versatile—great served with a sweet dessert wine or with a cold glass of milk. Any way you serve them, they won't last long!

2 cups	cake-and-pastry flour	500 mL
1/2 cup	soy flour	125 mL
1 cup	toasted chopped almonds	250 mL
1/2 cup	granulated sugar	125 mL
1 tsp	baking powder	5 mL
1/2 tsp	baking soda	2 mL
1/2 tsp	salt	2 mL
2	eggs	2
1/3 cup	liquid honey	75 mL
2 tbsp	imported orange liqueur or orange juice	25 mL
1 tbsp	grated orange rind	15 mL

Once cooled, this biscotti can be stored in a cookie tin at room temperature for up to 1 week. For longer storage, wrap well and freeze for up to 2 months.

1. Preheat oven to 325°F (160°C). Line baking sheet with parchment paper.
2. Sift together cake-and-pastry flour and soy flour into bowl. Stir in almonds, sugar, baking powder, baking soda and salt.
3. In separate bowl, whisk together eggs, honey, liqueur and orange rind.
4. Stir egg mixture into flour mixture until well mixed. Dough will be stiff.
5. Divide dough into 2 equal portions. Roll each portion into a 1-inch (2.5 cm) diameter log. Place on prepared baking sheet.
6. Bake in 325°F (160°C) oven for 40 to 50 minutes or until pale brown. Let cool.
7. Using sharp knife, slice logs on the diagonal at 1/2-inch (1 cm) intervals. Arrange slices on baking sheet. Bake in 350°F (180°C) oven for 10 minutes.

Per piece	
CALCIUM	22 mg
VITAMIN D	2 IU
Calories	89
Protein	3 g
Fat	3 g
Carbohydrate	14 g
Dietary Fiber	1 g
Sodium	72 mg
Magnesium	19 mg

Lactose-Free Shortbread

Slice and bake. What could be easier? Designed for the lactose-intolerant, but delicious for anyone, this shortbread gets calcium from the soy flour and sesame seeds.

Makes about 5 dozen

2 cups	**all-purpose flour**	**500 mL**
1/2 cup	**soy flour or all-purpose flour**	**125 mL**
1/2 tsp	**salt**	**2 mL**
1 cup	**shortening**	**250 mL**
3/4 cup	**packed brown sugar**	**175 mL**
2 tsp	**vanilla extract**	**10 mL**
1/4 cup	**sesame seeds**	**50 mL**

1. Line baking sheet with parchment paper.
2. In mixing bowl, stir together all-purpose flour, soy flour and salt.
3. In separate bowl, using electric mixer, beat together shortening, brown sugar and vanilla until fluffy. Gradually beat in flour mixture, 1/2 cup (125 mL) at a time, scraping down bowl occasionally.
4. Use a sheet of waxed paper to shape dough into log 1 1/2 inches (4 cm) in diameter. Sprinkle sesame seeds onto waxed paper. Roll log in sesame seeds to coat. Wrap tightly and refrigerate for 1 hour.
5. Preheat oven to 350°F (180°C). Using sharp knife, slice log at 1/4-inch (5 mm) intervals; arrange on prepared baking sheet.
6. Bake in 350°F (180°C) oven for 20 to 25 minutes or until golden brown. Shortbread may be stored in cookie tin at room temperature for up to 1 week. For longer storage, wrap well and freeze for up to 3 months.

Per piece	
CALCIUM	5 mg
Calories	62
Protein	1 g
Fat	4 g
Carbohydrate	6 g
Dietary Fiber	trace
Sodium	20 mg
Magnesium	6 mg

Light and Luscious Cheesecake

Makes 8 servings

As a cheesecake enthusiast, I have sampled many varieties. This recipe is still my favorite. It is rich without being overly cloying and it has that delectable bite of lemon, which is so enticing. For extra visual delight, you can top this off with fresh berries.

CRUST:

1 1/4 cups	graham cracker crumbs	300 mL
1/4 cup	ground almonds	50 mL
2 tbsp	granulated sugar	25 mL
1/2 tsp	cinnamon	2 mL
1/4 cup	melted butter	50 mL

FILLING:

1 cup	granulated sugar, divided	250 mL
1 tbsp	grated lemon rind	15 mL
2 cups	2% cottage cheese	500 mL
4	eggs, separated	4
1/2 cup	Drained Yogurt (p. 45) or yogurt	125 mL
1/4 cup	all-purpose flour	50 mL
2 tbsp	lemon juice	25 mL
1 tsp	vanilla extract	5 mL

TOPPING:

1 cup	All-Purpose Yogurt Dessert Sauce (p. 45)*	250 mL

*If time is tight, as an alternative to the All-Purpose Yogurt Dessert Sauce, stir together the following ingredients to use as a topping: 1 cup (250 mL) yogurt, 2 tbsp (25 mL) granulated sugar and 1 tsp (5 mL) vanilla extract.

1. Preheat oven to 350°F (180°C). Line bottom of 9-inch (2.5 L) springform pan with parchment paper.
2. Crust: In small bowl, combine graham cracker crumbs, almonds, sugar and cinnamon. Stir in melted butter. Press into bottom and partway up sides of prepared springform pan. Bake in 350°F (180°C) oven for 10 minutes. Let cool on rack. Reduce heat to 325°F (160°C).

Per serving	
CALCIUM	159 mg
VITAMIN D	18 IU
Calories	434
Protein	18 g
Fat	13 g
Carbohydrate	63 g
Dietary Fiber	1 g
Sodium	458 mg
Magnesium	30 mg

Scones with Cheddar Cheese (page 25), Almond Shortbread (page 136), Molasses Crinkles (page 138), Chocolate-Apricot Chews (page 137), Savory Cheddar and Orange Cheesecake (page 51), and Cranberry-Orange Chutney (page 43)

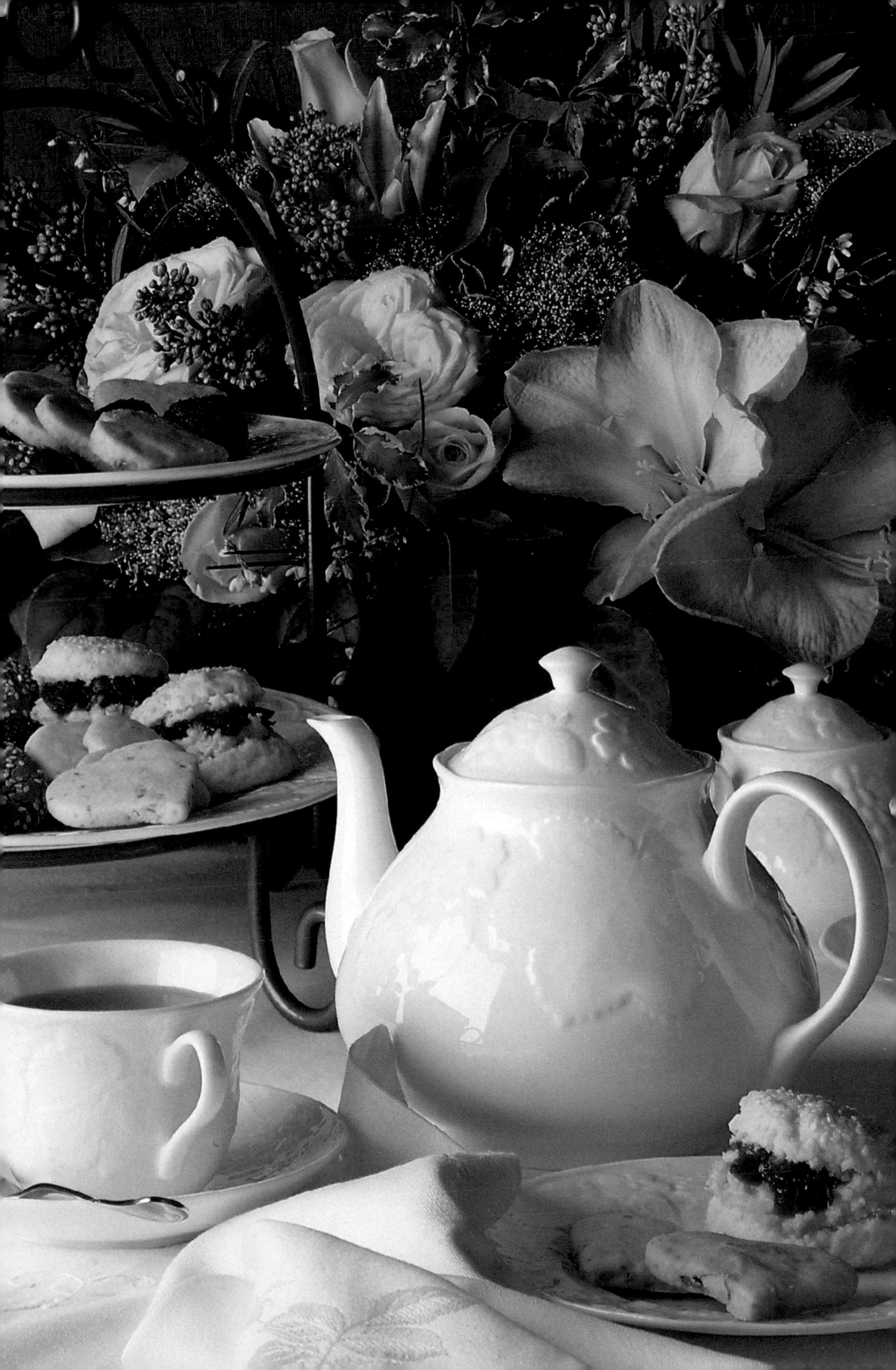

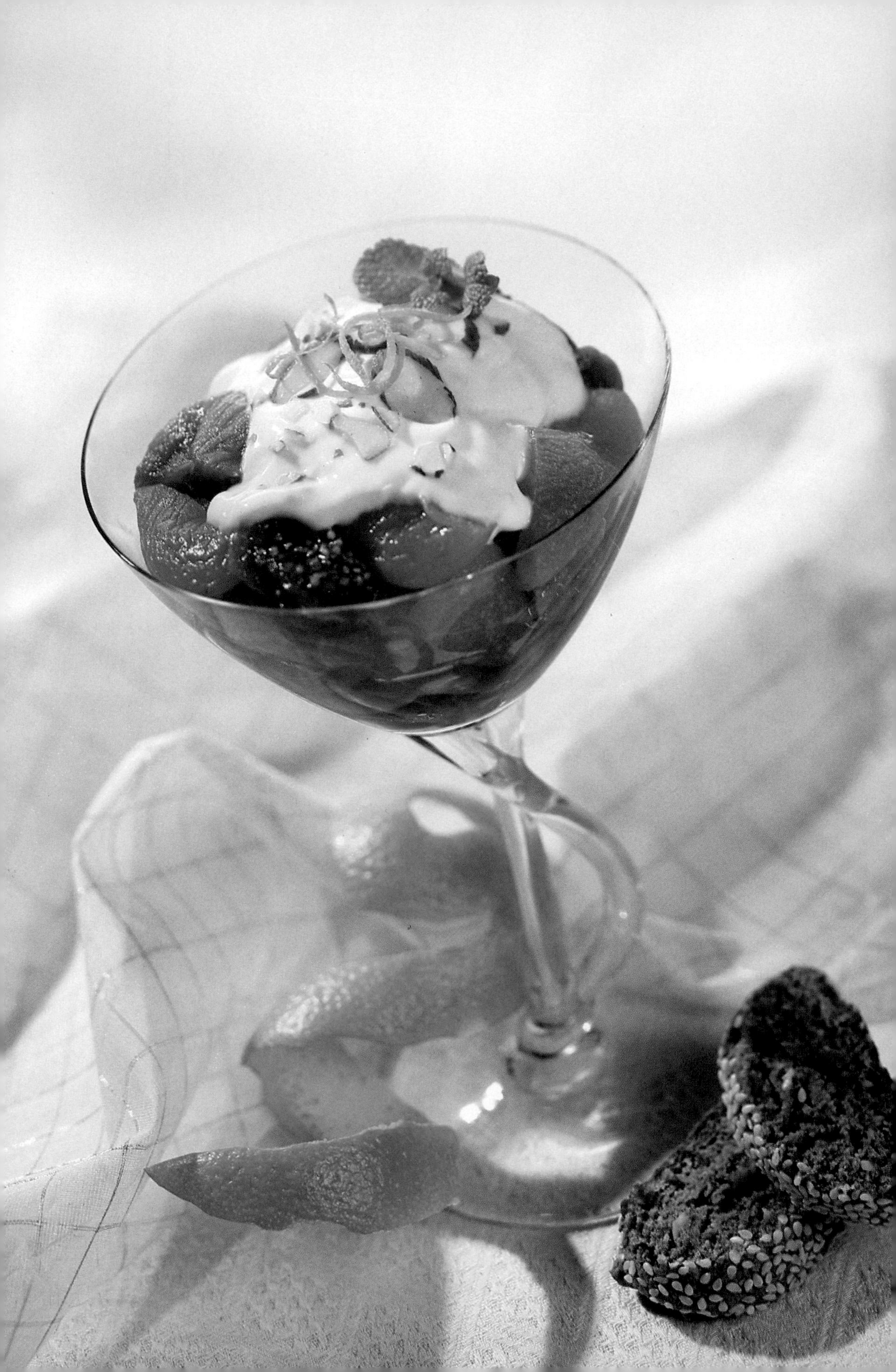

3. Filling: In food processor, combine 1/2 cup (125 mL) of the sugar and lemon rind. Add cottage cheese; process until smooth. Add egg yolks, drained yogurt, flour, lemon juice and vanilla; process until smooth. Transfer to large bowl.
4. In separate large bowl, beat egg whites until soft peaks form; gradually add remaining sugar, beating until stiff peaks form. Fold egg whites into egg yolk mixture.
5. Assembly: Spoon batter into crust. Bake in 325°F (160°C) oven for 1 1/4 hrs or until cheesecake is firm and golden brown around edge.
6. Let cool to room temperature on rack; cover and refrigerate. May be kept covered and refrigerated for up to 1 day.
7. Topping: Before serving, top with All-Purpose Yogurt Dessert Sauce.

Fig and Apricot Compote in Brandy (page 151) with Spectacular Spicy Biscotti (page 140)

Fig-Date Squares

Makes 16 servings

Serve this delectable square with a spoonful of All-Purpose Yogurt Dessert Sauce (p. 45) for a yummy calcium treat.

1 1/2 cups	quick-cooking rolled oats	375 mL
1 cup	all-purpose flour	250 mL
3/4 cup	packed brown sugar	175 mL
1/2 cup	soy flour	125 mL
1/4 cup	toasted chopped hazelnuts	50 mL
1/4 cup	toasted chopped almonds	50 mL
1 tsp	baking powder	5 mL
1/2 tsp	baking soda	2 mL
1 cup	melted butter or shortening	250 mL

FILLING:

3 cups	finely chopped dates (about 3/4 lb/375 g)	750 mL
2 1/2 cups	finely chopped dried figs (about 3/4 lb/375 g)	625 mL
1 1/2 cups	boiling water	375 mL
1/4 cup	orange juice	50 mL
2 tbsp	molasses	25 mL
1 tbsp	lemon juice	15 mL
1 tsp	grated orange rind	5 mL
1 tsp	vanilla extract	5 mL

1. Preheat oven to 350°F (180°C). Grease 13- x 9-inch (3.5 L) baking dish or spray with nonstick cooking spray.
2. In bowl, stir together oats, all-purpose flour, brown sugar, soy flour, hazelnuts, almonds, baking powder and baking soda. Stir in melted butter.

Per serving	
CALCIUM	81 mg
Calories	353
Protein	5 g
Fat	15 g
Carbohydrate	55 g
Dietary Fiber	6 g
Sodium	178 mg
Magnesium	57 mg

3. Press half of the oat mixture into bottom of prepared baking dish.
4. Filling: In large saucepan, combine dates, figs, water, orange juice, molasses, lemon juice, orange rind and vanilla. Cook over medium heat, stirring, for 5 to 10 minutes or until thickened.
5. Assembly: Spoon filling evenly over crumble base. Sprinkle remaining crumble over filling, pressing down gently.
6. Bake in 350°F (180°C) oven for 30 to 35 minutes or until golden brown. Let stand and cool before cutting into squares.

Sticky-Toffee Fig Pudding

Makes 8 servings

A wintry night is a great excuse to serve these festive, individual puddings. Hot, gooey and with all the buttery sweetness of toffee, they are lip-smacking good!

TOFFEE SAUCE:

1/4 cup	butter	50 mL
1/2 cup	packed brown sugar	125 mL
1 cup	2% evaporated milk	250 mL

PUDDING:

1/2 cup	boiling water	125 mL
1 cup	chopped dried figs	250 mL
1 tsp	instant coffee granules	5 mL
1 tsp	baking soda	5 mL
1 tsp	vanilla extract	5 mL
1 1/2 cups	cake-and-pastry flour	375 mL
2 tsp	baking powder	10 mL
1/2 tsp	salt	5 mL
1/3 cup	butter, softened	75 mL
1 cup	packed brown sugar	250 mL
2	eggs	2

TOPPING:

1/2 cup	toasted chopped almonds	125 mL

1. Toffee Sauce: In saucepan over medium-high heat, melt butter and sugar. Cook, stirring constantly, for 5 minutes. (Mixture will be smooth and thick.) Remove from heat. Carefully pour in 1/2 cup (125 mL) of the milk, stirring with long-handled spoon. (Mixture is very hot and steamy at this point.) Continue to stir until toffee sauce is smooth. Return to heat; gradually stir in remaining milk, stirring constantly until toffee sauce is smooth and thickened like cream, about 3 minutes. Sauce may be kept in jar in refrigerator for up to 2 days and reheated before serving.

Per serving	
CALCIUM	219 mg
VITAMIN D	32 IU
Calories	502
Protein	8 g
Fat	20 g
Carbohydrate	76 g
Dietary Fiber	4 g
Sodium	559 mg
Magnesium	60 mg

2. Pudding: Preheat oven to 350°F (180°C). Spray eight 3/4-cup (175 mL) ramekins with nonstick cooking spray; line each bottom with round of parchment paper. Put ramekins on baking sheet.
3. In small bowl, pour boiling water over figs. Stir in coffee granules, baking soda and vanilla; let stand.
4. Meanwhile, sift together flour, baking powder and salt.
5. In separate bowl, cream butter with brown sugar; add eggs, 1 at a time, beating well after each addition.
6. Beginning and ending with flour mixture, add flour mixture and fig mixture alternately to creamed butter mixture, combining well. Divide batter among prepared ramekins.
7. Bake in 350°F (180°C) oven for 25 to 30 minutes or until firm to touch and toothpick inserted in center comes away clean. Let cool for 10 minutes.
8. Assembly: Unmold each ramekin onto individual dessert plate. Top each with about 2 tbsp (25 mL) Toffee Sauce and 1 tbsp (15 mL) chopped almonds.

Gingerbread

Makes 8 servings

There are many versions of this classic treat, but if you like one that is moist and chewy with an extra zip of ginger, this one is for you! Cut into wedges and serve warm with a dollop of All-Purpose Yogurt Dessert Sauce (p. 45) or Frozen Lemon Yogurt (p. 156).

1/2 cup	**molasses**	**125 mL**
1/3 cup	**packed brown sugar**	**75 mL**
1/3 cup	**butter, softened**	**75 mL**
1/4 cup	**1% plain yogurt**	**50 mL**
1	**egg**	**1**
2 cups	**all-purpose flour**	**500 mL**
1 tbsp	**ground ginger**	**15 mL**
1 tsp	**cinnamon**	**5 mL**
1 tsp	**baking soda**	**5 mL**
1/4 tsp	**salt**	**1 mL**
3/4 cup	**mixed chopped dried apricots, figs and dates**	**175 mL**

1. Preheat oven to 350°F (180°C). Spray a 9-inch (1.5 L) round cake pan with nonstick cooking spray.
2. Using electric mixer, cream together molasses, brown sugar and butter until fluffy. Beat in yogurt and egg. (Mixture will look curdled.)
3. In separate bowl, stir together flour, ginger, cinnamon, baking soda and salt.
4. Stir flour mixture into yogurt mixture just until moistened. Fold in dried fruit.
5. Spoon into prepared pan. Bake in 350°F (180°C) oven for 45 minutes or until toothpick inserted in center comes out clean.

Per serving	
CALCIUM	73 mg
VITAMIN D	4 IU
Calories	321
Protein	5 g
Fat	9 g
Carbohydrate	57 g
Dietary Fiber	3 g
Sodium	315 mg
Magnesium	27 mg

Fig and Apricot Compote in Brandy

A luscious calcium finish to a brunch or rich evening meal, this "fruit salad" gets better as it mellows in the refrigerator.

Makes 6 servings

1 cup	dried figs, halved	250 mL
1 cup	dried apricots, halved	250 mL
1	orange	1
1/4 cup	granulated sugar	50 mL
1/2 cup	apricot brandy	125 mL

Use a stainless-steel saucepan so that acid from the fruit and juice does not react with the metal.

BRANDY CREAM SAUCE:

1	container (750 mL) 1% plain yogurt	1
2 tbsp	granulated sugar	25 mL
2 tbsp	apricot brandy	25 mL
1/3 cup	chopped toasted almonds or hazelnuts or mixture	75 mL

1. In mixing bowl, pour enough boiling water to cover over figs and apricots. Let stand for about 5 minutes. Drain.
2. In stainless-steel saucepan, combine figs, apricots, grated rind of the orange, squeezed juice from the orange and sugar. Add enough water to cover fruit. Bring to boil. Reduce heat; simmer for 5 to 10 minutes. Remove from heat. Let cool for about 15 minutes. Pour into serving bowl; stir in apricot brandy. Cover and refrigerate until chilled, about 4 hours or overnight.
4. Brandy Cream Sauce: Meanwhile, line sieve with cheesecloth or coffee filter; drain yogurt for at least 3 hours or overnight. Keep covered and refrigerated. Stir sugar and apricot brandy into drained yogurt. Spoon into serving bowl.
5. Assembly: Sprinkle nuts over chilled fruit compote. To serve, spoon compote into individual serving bowls and accompany with Brandy Cream Sauce.

Per serving	
CALCIUM	196 mg
Calories	369
Protein	9 g
Fat	5 g
Carbohydrate	65 g
Dietary Fiber	6 g
Sodium	41 mg
Magnesium	55 mg

Orange-Almond Cake

Makes 16 servings

You could not ask for an easier, more delicious cake to serve for coffee or dessert; simply mix the batter in one bowl and pour into a pan ready to bake.

3	eggs	3
2 cups	granulated sugar	500 mL
3/4 cup	vegetable oil	175 mL
1 tbsp	grated orange rind	15 mL
1 tsp	almond extract	5 mL
1 1/2 cups	all-purpose flour	375 mL
1/2 cup	soy flour	125 mL
2 tsp	baking powder	10 mL
1/2 tsp	salt	2 mL
1/2 cup	chopped dates	125 mL
1/2 cup	toasted sliced almonds	125 mL

ORANGE-ALMOND GLAZE:

1/2 cup	orange juice	125 mL
1/3 cup	granulated sugar	75 mL
1/4 tsp	almond extract	1 mL

To toast almonds, place nuts on baking sheet; bake in 350°F (180°C) oven for about 15 minutes or until almonds are golden brown and fragrant.

1. Preheat oven to 350°F (180°C). Spray 9-inch (3 L) bundt pan with nonstick cooking spray.
2. In mixing bowl, using electric mixer, beat eggs until foamy. Gradually beat in sugar until thick and creamy.
3. Gradually beat in oil until thick. Beat in orange rind and almond extract.
4. Beat in all-purpose flour, soy flour, baking powder and salt until combined.
5. Using spatula, fold in dates and almonds.

Per serving	
CALCIUM	37 mg
VITAMIN D	6 IU
Calories	306
Protein	4 g
Fat	13 g
Carbohydrate	45 g
Dietary Fiber	1 g
Sodium	117 mg
Magnesium	23 mg

6. Pour batter into prepared pan. Bake in 350°F (180°C) oven for 45 to 50 minutes or until toothpick inserted in center comes away clean.
7. Orange-Almond Glaze: Meanwhile, in saucepan, bring orange juice and sugar to boil. Boil for 2 minutes. Remove from heat; stir in almond extract.
8. Assembly: Let cake cool on rack for 15 minutes. Run knife around edge; invert cake onto serving plate. Drizzle Orange-Almond Glaze evenly over cake. Glazed cake keeps well for up to 3 days in refrigerator. For longer storage, wrap and freeze cake for up to 3 months.

Pavlova

Makes 6 servings

One of the best-loved cream-filled meringue desserts, this slimmed-down Pavlova makes the most of low-fat yogurt and almonds to create a scrumptious version that's lower in fat and higher in calcium than the original.

Eggs are easier to separate when cold, straight from the refrigerator. However, separated egg whites that are at room temperature will whip to a greater volume than cold egg whites.

Even a speck of yolk will prevent the whites from whipping to maximum volume. To ensure yolk-free whites, use three bowls when separating eggs: one to separate eggs over; one to transfer the uncontaminated whites into; and one for the yolks.

ALMOND-YOGURT FILLING:

1	container (750 g) 1% plain yogurt	1
1/4 cup	granulated sugar	50 mL
1 tsp	almond extract	5 mL

MERINGUE:

4	egg whites	4
1/2 tsp	cream of tartar	2 mL
1 cup	granulated sugar	250 mL
2 tbsp	cornstarch	25 mL
1 tsp	vanilla extract	5 mL
1/2 cup	toasted sliced almonds, divided	125 mL

FRUIT TOPPING:

6	ripe peaches, sliced or a 14 oz (398 mL) can unsweetened sliced peaches packed in juice, drained	6

1. Almond-Yogurt Filling: Line sieve with cheesecloth or single thickness of coffee filters. Spoon yogurt into sieve; let drain for 3 hours or overnight, covered, in refrigerator.
2. In bowl, stir together drained yogurt, sugar and almond extract until smooth. Cover and refrigerate until ready to use.
3. Meringue: Preheat oven to 300°F (150°C). Using 9-inch (23 cm) plate as template, draw and cut out 9-inch (23 cm) circle of parchment paper; arrange circle on baking sheet.

Per serving	
CALCIUM	150 mg
Calories	326
Protein	10 g
Fat	5 g
Carbohydrate	61 g
Dietary Fiber	2 g
Sodium	71 mg
Magnesium	42 mg

4. In mixing bowl, using electric mixer, beat egg whites and cream of tartar until soft peaks form. Gradually beat in sugar, a spoonful at a time, until stiff peaks form. Fold in cornstarch and vanilla.
5. Spoon meringue onto parchment circle, smoothing to within 1 inch (2.5 cm) of the edge. Using back of dampened spoon, indent center, sweeping all the way outward and upward with spoon to make a bowl with peaked edges. Sprinkle meringue with 1/4 cup (50 mL) of the almonds.
6. Bake in 300°F (150°C) oven for 35 minutes or until pale golden brown. Turn oven off; let meringue cool completely in oven.
7. Assembly: Gently remove parchment from meringue; discard parchment. Place meringue on serving plate. Spoon Almond-Yogurt Filling into center. Arrange peach slices decoratively on yogurt. Sprinkle with remaining almonds.

Leftover egg yolks may be used in recipes to make ice cream, custard, scrambled eggs and rice puddings.

Make-ahead: The yogurt needs a minimum of 3 hours to drain. Or, drain it overnight. The meringue shell may be made up to 1 day ahead.

Frozen Lemon Yogurt

Makes about 2 cups (500 mL)

This versatile recipe should be in everyone's repertoire. Serve this frozen yogurt as a sauce for fruit or cake; serve it semifreddo as a frozen dessert; or serve it as a filling for Pavlova or tartlets. It is simple, stylish and scrumptious!

1	**container (750 g) 1% plain yogurt**	**1**
1 cup	**granulated sugar**	**250 mL**
1/2 cup	**fresh lemon juice**	**125 mL**
1 tbsp	**grated lemon rind**	**15 mL**
2	**eggs**	**2**

Use a stainless-steel saucepan so that the acid in the lemon juice will not react with the metal.

1. Line sieve with cheesecloth or 2 coffee filters. Place sieve over bowl. Spoon in yogurt. Cover and refrigerate for at least 1 hour or overnight.
2. In stainless-steel saucepan over medium heat, whisk together sugar, lemon juice, rind and eggs until smooth. Continue to cook, whisking frequently, until lemon mixture thickens and coats back of spoon, about 5 to 8 minutes.
3. Remove from heat. Let cool.
4. When cool, fold lemon mixture into drained yogurt.
5. To use as frozen yogurt, freeze mixture; thaw in refrigerator for 20 minutes before serving.

VARIATION:
To use as a filling or a sauce for cake, fruit or desserts, use lemon-yogurt mixture at room temperature. Keep in a covered container for up to 1 week in refrigerator. For longer storage, freeze for up to 1 month.

Per 1/2 cup (125 mL)	
CALCIUM	201 mg
VITAMIN D	18 IU
Calories	322
Protein	12 g
Fat	4 g
Carbohydrate	61 g
Dietary Fiber	trace
Sodium	82 mg
Magnesium	20 mg

Cheater's Banana Ice Cream

A very banana "ice cream," this super-simple version really cheats as ice cream because it contains no cream. The creamy texture comes from puréed bananas and 2% evaporated milk.

Makes about 2 1/2 cups (625 mL), 4 servings

3	**ripe bananas**	**3**
1/2 cup	**granulated sugar**	**125 mL**
1 cup	**2% evaporated milk**	**250 mL**
2 tsp	**vanilla extract**	**10 mL**

1. In food processor, purée bananas and sugar until smooth. With motor running, pour in milk and vanilla.
2. Freeze according to ice-cream machine directions. (Alternatively, spoon purée into shallow container; freeze for at least 4 hours.) Serve within 24 hours for best texture.

Per serving	
CALCIUM	180 mg
VITAMIN D	55 IU
Calories	241
Protein	6 g
Fat	2 g
Carbohydrate	53 g
Dietary Fiber	1 g
Sodium	71 mg
Magnesium	41 mg

Freezer Strawberry Ice Cream

You can quickly transform frozen strawberries into a luscious frozen dessert. It is ready so quickly, you need to have everything prepared for serving.

Makes 4 servings

4 cups	**frozen strawberries**	**1 L**
1/2 cup	**granulated sugar**	**125 mL**
1	**can (385 mL) 2% evaporated milk**	**1**
1 tsp	**vanilla extract**	**5 mL**

1. In food processor, purée strawberries and sugar until smooth. With motor running, pour milk and vanilla through feed tube.
2. "Ice cream" may be frozen enough to serve immediately. If not, use ice-cream maker to finish off freezing. (Alternatively, spoon mixture into shallow pan; freeze for about 1 hour or until firm but not hard.)

Per serving	
CALCIUM	309 mg
VITAMIN D	90 IU
Calories	246
Protein	8 g
Fat	2 g
Carbohydrate	50 g
Dietary Fiber	2 g
Sodium	118 mg
Magnesium	43 mg

Any-Fruit Crisp

Makes 6 servings

Change this popular dessert with seasonal fruit: peaches in the summer; strawberries and rhubarb in the spring; and cranberries and apples in the fall. Any way you bake it, the dessert is guaranteed to disappear! By using soy flour, almonds and dried figs, the crisp has been enriched with calcium. If you serve it with All-Purpose Yogurt Dessert Sauce (p. 45), Freezer Strawberry Ice Cream (p. 157) or Frozen Lemon Yogurt (p. 156), you have made a contribution to daily calcium.

FRUIT FILLING:

1/3 cup	granulated sugar	75 mL
2 tbsp	soy flour	25 mL
1/2 tsp	cinnamon	2 mL
4 1/2 cups	sliced fruit (fresh or frozen)	1.25 L
1/2 cup	chopped dried figs or dates or raisins	125 mL

TOPPING:

3/4 cup	quick-cooking rolled oats	175 mL
1/3 cup	packed brown sugar	75 mL
1/4 cup	soy flour	50 mL
1/4 cup	chopped almonds	50 mL
1 tsp	cinnamon	5 mL
1/4 tsp	salt	1 mL
1/4 cup	melted butter	50 mL

1. Preheat oven to 375°F (190°C). Grease 6-cup (1.5 L) baking dish or spray with nonstick cooking spray.
2. Fruit Filling: In large bowl, combine sugar, soy flour and cinnamon. Gently fold in fruit and figs.

Per serving	
CALCIUM	93 mg
Calories	376
Protein	8 g
Fat	15 g
Carbohydrate	59 g
Dietary Fiber	6 g
Sodium	182 mg
Magnesium	101 mg

3. Spoon fruit filling into prepared baking dish. Set aside.
4. Topping: In mixing bowl, combine oats, brown sugar, soy flour, almonds, cinnamon and salt. Stir in melted butter.
5. Assembly: Spoon topping over fruit filling. Bake in 375°F (190°C) oven for 40 to 50 minutes, until fruit filling is bubbling and topping is brown. (Frozen fruit filling will take longer to cook than fresh fruit filling.) Serve warm or at room temperature. Baked crisps may be wrapped well and frozen for up to 2 months.

Almond-Hazelnut Roulade with Ricotta Filling

Makes 8 servings

A truly elegant dessert for a special occasion, the roulade can be filled with the ricotta filling or, as a lactose-free alternative, spread with apricot jam flavored with rum.

1/2 cup	unblanched almonds	125 mL
1/2 cup	unblanched hazelnuts	125 mL
1/4 cup	all-purpose flour	50 mL
1 tsp	baking powder	5 mL
5	eggs, separated	5
2/3 cup	granulated sugar, divided	150 mL
1/4 tsp	cream of tartar	1 mL
1/4 tsp	salt	1 mL
	Sifted icing sugar	
	Ricotta-Apricot Filling or Frosting (p. 48)	
8	unblanched almonds or hazelnuts	8

1. Preheat oven to 350°F (180°C). Line 15- x 10-inch (2 L) jelly roll pan with parchment paper.
2. On separate baking sheets, toast almonds and hazelnuts in 350°F (180°C) oven for about 15 minutes or until fragrant. When cool enough to handle, rub hazelnuts in tea towel to remove skins. In food processor, chop almonds, hazelnuts, flour and baking powder until nuts are finely chopped.
3. In separate bowl, beat egg yolks with 1/3 cup (75 mL) of the sugar for about 3 minutes or until pale and thickened. Fold in nut mixture.

Per serving	
CALCIUM	202 mg
VITAMIN D	22 IU
Calories	393
Protein	14 g
Fat	22 g
Carbohydrate	36 g
Dietary Fiber	2 g
Sodium	196 mg
Magnesium	72 mg

4. In separate bowl, beat egg whites with cream of tartar and salt until soft peaks form. Gradually beat in remaining sugar until stiff peaks form. Fold about one-quarter of the egg white mixture into yolk-nut mixture. Gently fold in remaining egg whites.
5. Spoon mixture onto prepared jelly roll pan, spreading smoothly. Bake in 350°F (180°C) oven for 15 to 18 minutes, until golden brown. Let cool for about 10 minutes. Invert onto tea towel covered with sifted icing sugar. Using tea towel, roll roulade from short end. Let cool in tea towel for at least 1 hour or overnight.
6. Gently unroll cake. Spread all but 1/2 cup (125 mL) of the ricotta filling on surface of cake. Gently reroll cake without tea towel; using spatulas, transfer roulade to serving platter. Using remaining ricotta filling, make 8 decorative rosettes along top surface of roulade. Place an almond in center of each rosette. With sharp knife, cut roulade into 8 slices. Roulade keeps well for up to 2 days, covered and refrigerated.

Exercises

Exercises

Move Those Bones

Bone is living tissue, constantly changing throughout our lives as old bone is replaced by new bone. This process is called remodelling and can be described this way: bone-eroding cells called *osteoclasts* invade the bone's surface and dissolve the mineral, forming small cavities in the bone's surface. Once the erosion is complete, bone-building cells called *osteoblasts* begin to fill in the cavities with new bone to restore the surface.

PEAK BONE MASS

These two processes of bone remodelling, eroding and rebuilding, occur at about the same speed until somewhere between ages 20 and 30 when our bones have achieved peak bone mass. Peak bone mass is a term which means our bones have achieved their maximum strength and density. Once peak bone mass is reached, the rebuilding process slows down. New bone is not laid down as quickly as old bone is eroded. As a result, our bones gradually become thinner and more fragile. If the bones become so fragile and brittle that they fracture easily, this condition is called osteoporosis. Physical activity is an important aspect in the prevention of osteoporosis because it builds bone mass in young adult years and reduces our rate of bone loss in later years.

WE NEED TO BE ACTIVE

Just as adequate nutrition is essential for a healthy body, so is exercise critical for a healthy skeleton. Physical activity is defined as any body movement produced by the action of our muscles. Those people who are physically active have a lower incidence of such chronic disease as heart disease and diabetes.

They sleep better, they have more energy and generally feel better. In addition, they lower their risk of osteoporosis because bones require the stimulation of exercise to increase bone mass. Dr. Robert Faulkner, Professor and Dean, College of Physical Education, University of Saskatchewan, Saskatoon, says, "There is increasing evidence that bone-loading is an important, if not the most important, functional influence on bone mass and bone architecture." This bone-loading is explained by Dr. Raphael Chow of Queen Elizabeth Hospital, Toronto, as "the pull of muscle on the bone and force of gravity that creates electrical charges in the bone tissue which together result in the stimulation of bone formation." Our bones respond to increased load, that is, weight-bearing physical activity, by increasing in mass. If there is no physical activity, the bones will decrease in bone mass in response to the reduced load. This decrease in bone mass can be seen in astronauts who lose bone in their feet and hands while they're in space because they are not working against the force of gravity. However, their wrists, which they use more in space, do not lose bone mass.

LIFESTYLE AND EXERCISE

There was a time, not long ago, when getting enough exercise was not a problem. Children walked or rode their bicycles to and from school. After school, if not doing chores, they played games outside. In the past, adults were required to do more physical work at home and on the job because there was not the mechanization of today. Now, however, many people walk from their house to the car for a drive to work. Once at work, the job is often sedentary, sitting at a desk or computer. Similarly, children are frequently driven to school either by parents, school bus or public transportation. Like adults, much of the school day is spent sitting at a desk with little opportunity for physical exercise. Although after-school activities may include sports, many children go home to sit in front of the television or computer for entertainment. Despite all this "inactivity," for many of us, life is so frantic there is little time for exercise. We must realize how essential exercise is to our health and build it into our lives every day.

An active lifestyle must begin in childhood. This is especially important because children have a greater capacity to add new bone mass to their skeletons than adults do. During childhood and puberty, children have the opportunity to put mineral matter into the bone bank for their adult years, and reduce the risk of fracture as they age. Between ages 20 and 30, young adults achieve their peak bone mass; that is, bones reach their maximum strength and density. In healthy individuals, peak bone mass will remain stable for several years, then start to decrease. As discussed before, this loss occurs because, as we age, new bone is not laid down at the same rate as old bone is lost. (Generally, we lose about .5%–1% of bone a year, but the rate of loss increases dramatically for women after menopause because of the loss of the hormone estrogen.) As parents we need to encourage daily exercise and set an example for our children by showing that an active way of life promotes a healthy body. High peak bone mass in young people is the best protection against osteoporosis in later life. This is not to say that once you're over 30, it's too late to build healthy bones. At any age, bone will respond to increased physical activity.

Physical activity is necessary to:

- optimize peak bone mass in the growing years;
- maintain peak mass during adult years;
- maintain bone or decrease the rate of bone loss in older adult years; and
- decrease the risk of falling in older adult years by improving balance.

EXERCISE IS FUN

If the word "exercise" turns you off, don't use it. For many people, that term implies boring, repetitious work. For greater motivation, think "fun." For children, exercise consists of the games they love playing: tag, skipping, baseball, swimming, hockey, skating, hide-and-go-seek. Encourage them to play these games. On occasion join in their fun. Make sure that activities happen daily, with you or with friends. This sets the stage for a lifetime of happy, physical activity and physical well-being.

Just as we must encourage our children to do regular fun activities, you must also choose enjoyable activities for yourself and do them regularly. Whatever you do, it should be fun!

BONE-BUILDING EXERCISE

While physical activity is important for maintaining peak bone mass, certain kinds of exercise are better than others. Bone responds to weight-bearing activities that require you to support your body weight. Walking is one example of weight-bearing exercise. Other activities that fit this category include dancing, gardening, playing tennis, skiing, golfing, bicycling, playing baseball, playing hockey and, of course, participating in structured fitness classes. All of these activities not only involve the muscles but apply weight or stress to the bone, which promotes bone formation and a healthy skeleton.

Remember, too, that exercise is site specific, that is, if your exercise involves a specific part of your body, only those bones will be affected—for example, if you play tennis, the bones in your tennis arm will be strengthened the most. It is important to include activities for all parts of the body, especially the spine, wrist and hip areas which are particularly vulnerable to osteoporosis.

Although our hectic lifestyles often make it difficult to find time for daily exercise, walking is perhaps the easiest bone-building exercise to incorporate. Try the following suggestions:

- if possible, walk to work;
- park your car an extra distance from the office and walk;
- bypass the elevator and take the stairs;
- instead of taking the car to do an errand, take your bones for a walk;
- if you have to sit for most of the day at work, get up regularly and take a brief walk;
- walk the children to school; or
- walk the dog.

The Osteoporosis Society of Canada has walking tapes and an exercise video available to assist your fitness program; to order, call 1-800-463-6842.

Another type of exercise of great benefit to the bones is resistance exercise such as weight training, which involves repeatedly moving an object or your own body weight. Resistance exercise also develops muscles, co-ordination and balance, which are helpful in reducing the risk of falls.

Swimming, on the other hand, is an example of a non-weight-bearing activity. Although it is an excellent exercise for muscular strength, endurance and stretching, because the water supports your body, the muscles' pull and contraction puts only indirect stress on the bone. Swimming does not increase bone mass, but in combination with weight-bearing activity it can be a worthwhile part of an exercise program.

Many people find that a fitness class several times a week works well for them in combination with other activities. A fitness program can provide structure, a social setting and a leader who helps motivate and guide you. This makes the program more enjoyable, and perhaps easier to maintain than solo efforts.

If you are considering a fitness program, here are some guidelines:

- check that the instructors are qualified professionals who are certified by organizations such as the Canadian Society of Exercise Physiology (C.S.E.P.) or Provincial Fitness Councils;
- ask members about the reputation of the fitness program and the instructors;

- ask to observe at least one free class before enrolling to see if the program suits your needs and look for the following:
    - Is the facility clean, well ventilated and well lit?
    - Is the floor a resilient, user-friendly surface?
    - Does the club have the necessary equipment?
    - How does the instructor relate to students?
    - Can the instructor see everyone?
    - Are questions answered?
    - Is there a stress on safety and working at your own pace?
    - Have there been injuries?
    - Are exercises explained?
    - Is there a warm-up and cool-down?
- if you have heart problems, high blood pressure, muscular pain or breathing problems, check with your doctor before starting an exercise program.

Exercise is one important factor in bone health. It is our responsibility to "Be Bone Wise and Exercise." —Dr. Robert Faulkner.

BONE-SAVING HABITS

Life-long habits of good posture while sleeping, sitting, standing and walking will reduce back strain and prevent injuries. By slouching while sitting or standing, you put extra strain on the vertebrae in your back. Likewise, if you bend incorrectly, you put extra pressure on your spine. You want to do everything possible to keep the vertebrae in an aligned position for a strong, straight back.

Lying
Use a firm mattress with a pillow thick enough to keep your head in line with your spine. Your head should not be pushed up and forward. If you are lying on your side, avoid curling into a ball; instead, lie with your neck and back in line. You may need a firm pillow behind your back for support and a pillow between your knees for some extra comfort.

Getting Out of Bed

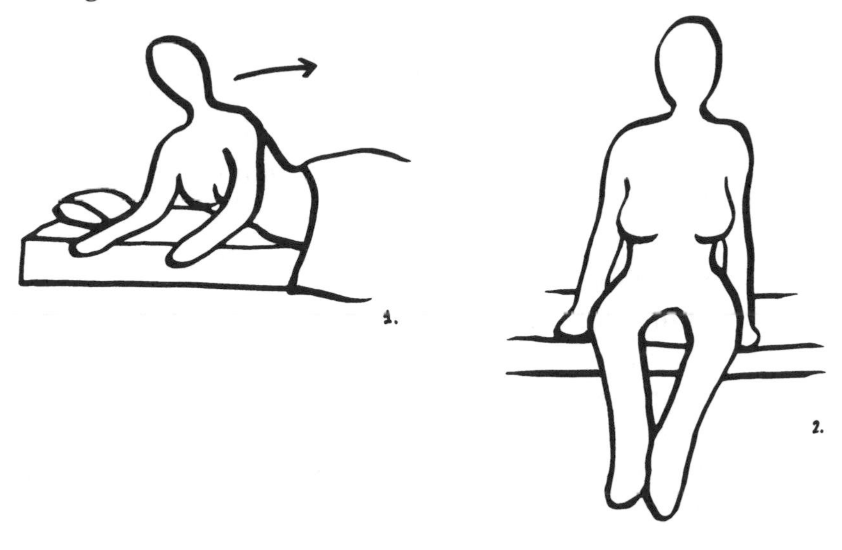

Roll onto your side and face the edge of the bed, keep your spine straight and use both hands to push yourself up into a sitting position without bending forward.

Getting Into Bed

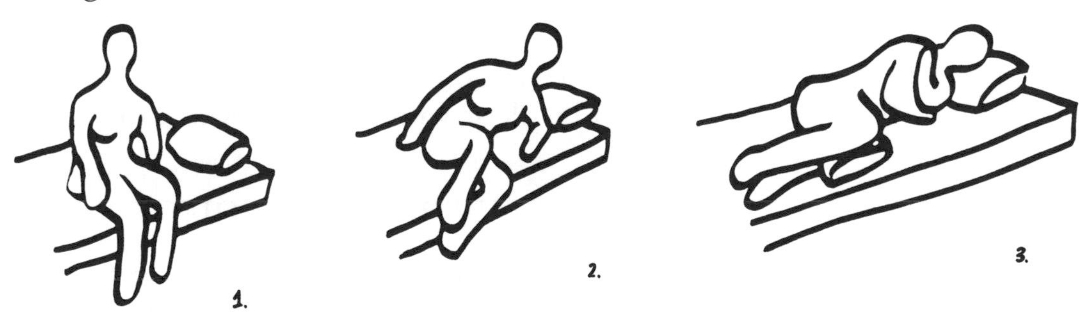

Sit on the side of the bed and use your arms to lower yourself down onto your side as you bring your legs up onto the bed.

Sitting

Sit erect in a firm chair that allows your feet to comfortably touch the floor. If the seat is too high, use a foot stool. If the seat is too deep, use a cushion for back support. To avoid pressure on your bones, do not slouch while sitting.

Sitting at Work—Reading, Writing, Typing or Driving
Again, sit erect with good back support and your feet on the floor. Sit facing your work and keep it (or the steering wheel) close enough to avoid either straining to reach it or contracting your muscles because it is too close.

Standing
Stand tall with your head erect, legs slightly apart, shoulders back, buttocks tucked under you with your abdominal muscles pulled in to support your lower back. This allows you to breathe easily while having a straight spine. Don't stand with your weight more on one hip than the other. Instead, stand with your weight on both feet and equally shared over both hips.

Getting Down to the Floor
Standing tall, slowly bend from your hips and slide your hands down onto your knees. Slowly bend your knees until your hands can comfortably reach the floor and then slowly lower your body down onto your knees. If you want to get onto your back, roll onto your bottom and gently ease your back down to the floor with the support of your arms.

THE BONE-BUILDING WORKOUT

A good exercise program includes stretching (for flexibility), endurance (for a cardiovascular workout) and strength (for muscle tone and bone-building).

Stretching: 10 minutes
Warm-ups and cool-downs are essential to an exercise program. They allow your muscles to relax and loosen up. The warm-up or stretching exercises in this section can be used in a cool-down period too. Select 10 minutes of exercise from the following choices. Vary your selections from time to time.

Safety Guidelines Before Exercise

- Consult your doctor before starting an exercise program if you have a heart condition, high blood pressure, arthritis or if you have been inactive for some time. These conditions may hinder your ability to perform the exercises safely.
- Exercise should not cause pain; if something hurts, stop the activity!
- Exercise should not cause shortness of breath.
- Wear comfortable, loose clothing and shoes with good support.
- Fatigue is normal after exercise.
- Some minor muscular soreness is normal after the first few exercise sessions but should go away after these initial sessions.
- Use a mat, if it would make you more comfortable.

The suggested number of repetitions is only a guideline. Our recommendations are conservative; let your fitness level be your guide as you gradually build your program.

1. Shoulder Shrug
Standing tall with your legs slightly apart, bring your shoulders up to your ears and down again. Repeat about 8–10 times. A great way to loosen up.

2. Flexibility
Standing tall, gently grasp the side of your head with one hand while your other hand reaches behind your back. Gently pull your head away until a gentle stretch is felt. Hold 10–30 seconds, depending on your comfort level. Repeat 3 times on each side.

3. Proper Standing Exercise
Standing tall with your back against the wall, hold your arms up with your elbows bent so that both

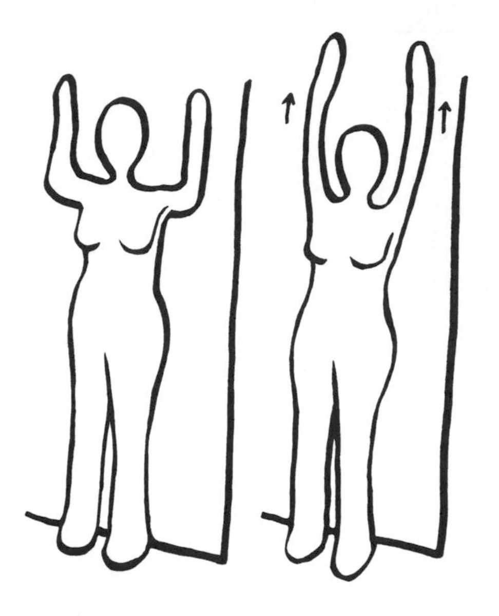

arms rest against the wall. Slowly slide your arms overhead, keeping them in touch with the wall as you straighten your arms. With your arms overhead, try to pull your abdomen up and in so that your back flattens against the wall. Try to keep your back flat against the wall as you slide your arms back down to the starting position.

4. Chest Stretch
Standing tall, intertwine the fingers of both hands behind your back and squeeze your shoulder blades together. Then slowly raise and straighten your arms. Hold 15–30 seconds, depending on your comfort level. Repeat 3 times.

5. Body Sway Variations

a) Standing tall with your feet slightly apart and knees slightly bent, sway to the right, then to the left. While slowly raising your arms from your sides to shoulder height, bring your elbows in and out, to the front, then to the side. Repeat 3 times.

b) Do the body sway with your arms at your sides, bending your arms until your fingers come up to touch your shoulders. Repeat 3 times.

c) While still doing the body sway, touch your shoulders with your finger tips, then bring both arms straight up over your head in a stretch. Repeat 3 times, then lower your arms back to your sides.

6. Arm Stretches
Standing tall with your palms facing in and your arms at your sides, slowly reach one arm up as far as it will go, stretching all your muscles on that side with the reach. Breathe in as your arm goes up and breathe out as your arm comes down. Repeat with your other arm. Repeat 8–10 times on each side. This is great for lung expansion.

7. Forward Shoulder Stretch
Standing tall, grasp your right elbow with your left hand; use your right hand to grasp your left shoulder blade. Hold 15–30 seconds, depending on your comfort level. Repeat on the other side. Repeat on each side 3 times.

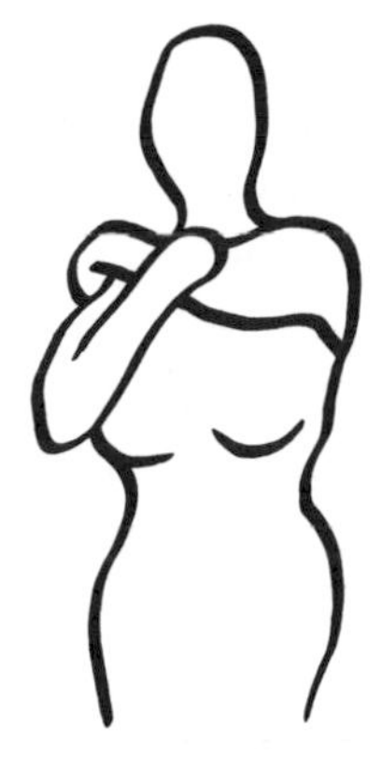

8. Backward Shoulder Stretch
Standing tall, put your right arm behind your head and use your left hand to reach back and grasp your right elbow. Try to touch your right hand to your left shoulder blade. Hold 15–30 seconds, depending on your comfort level. Repeat on the other side. Repeat 3 times on each side.

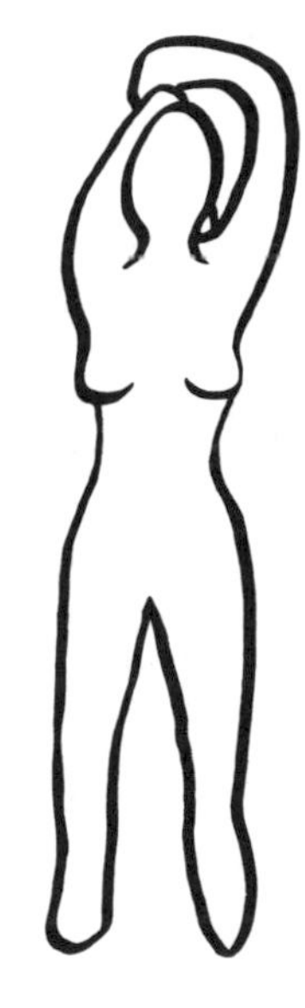

9. Loosen-up Swing
Standing tall with your knees relaxed, swing your arms from side to side for 30–60 seconds.

10. Hand Stretches
Standing tall with your arms in front at shoulder height, grip your hands together. Push your hands forward with your palms outward and your fingers entwined; then pull fingers of each hand back as far as they will go, first your left hand, then your right. Repeat 3–4 times with each hand. This is a great exercise to loosen up your hands if you spend a lot of time inputting.

11. Thigh Stretches for Balance
Standing tall and keeping your back flat against the wall, bring your knee up as far as possible. Hold for 15–30 seconds, then slowly lower your foot to the floor. You will feel the stretch in your straight leg. Alternate legs, repeating the exercise 3 times.

12. Thigh Stengthening Exercise
Stand tall about a foot from a wall, with your back to the wall and your feet set shoulder-width apart. Lean back and use your arms to help you slide down the wall until your knees are at a 30 to 45 degree angle; keep your back flat against the wall and hold the position until thigh muscle fatigue sets in (about 15 seconds). Use your arms to help you return to your original position. Repeat up to 5 times as you build your thigh strength.

13. Hamstring Stretch

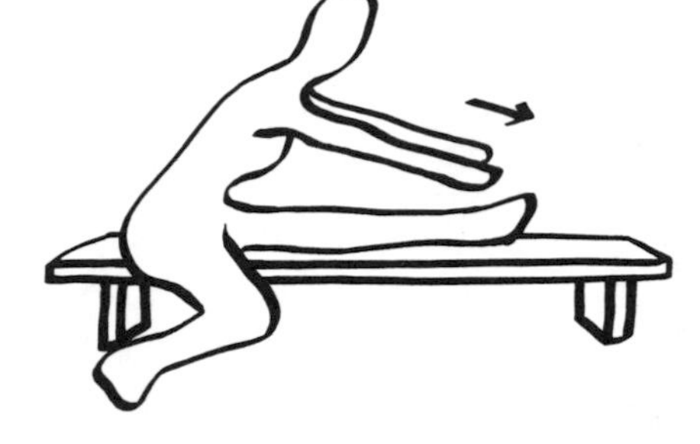

Sit lengthwise along a bench, bed or sofa with one foot on the floor and one leg straightened along the top of the bench. Keep your back straight. Lean forward from your hips, reaching your fingers toward your toes until a stretch is felt at the back of your thigh. Hold 15–30 seconds, depending on your comfort level. Repeat 3 times and then switch to the other side.

14. Body Sways with One Knee Bent
Stand tall with your arms hanging loosely at your sides and your legs apart. Sway to the right, bending your right knee while keeping your left leg straight. Sway to the left with your left knee bent and your right leg straight. Repeat 5 times in each direction.

The following exercises are done on the floor. Consult "Getting Down to the Floor" on page 172 for the safest way to get to the floor. Use a mat (or a thick towel) if you would be more comfortable.

15. Stretching Legs on All Fours
Get down on all fours, keeping your back flat. Support your upper body with your arms and, without arching your neck or your back, raise one leg behind you, keeping your knee slightly flexed. Raise your leg no more than 90 to 100 degrees. Hold for 5 seconds. Slowly lower your leg and repeat on the other side. Repeat 5 times with each leg.

16. Trunk Forward Lean

Get down on all fours, keeping your back flat and supporting your upper body with your arms. Tighten your stomach muscles as you slowly lean forward. Hold for 10 seconds. Repeat 5 times.

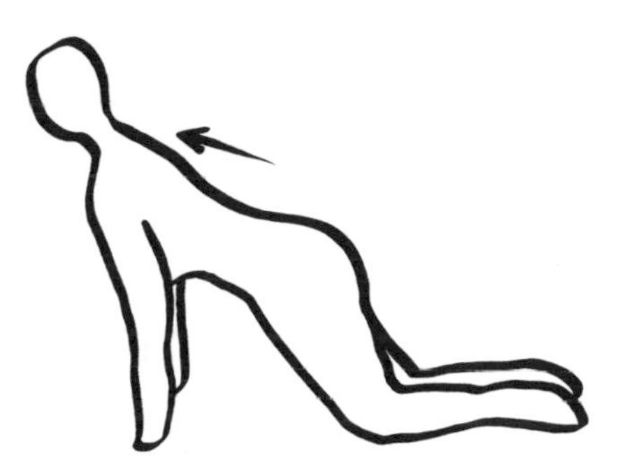

17. Trunk Stability with One Arm Extended

Get down on all fours, supporting your upper body with your arms. Tighten your stomach muscles as you raise one arm parallel to the floor. Hold for 5 seconds, then slowly return to your starting position, keeping your trunk rigid. Repeat 10 times, alternating sides.

18. Trunk Stability

Get down on all fours, supporting your upper body with your arms. Tighten your stomach muscles and simultaneously raise your right leg and your left arm. Hold for 15–30 seconds, depending on your comfort level, then slowly return to your starting position, keeping your back flat. Repeat with your left leg and your right arm, 5 times on each side.

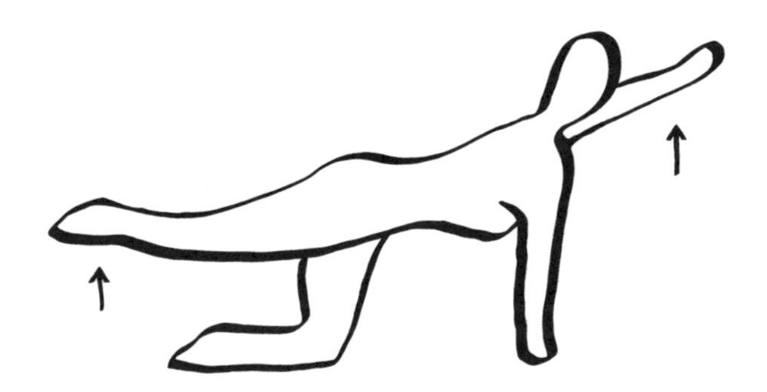

19. Cat Stretch

Get down on all fours, supporting your upper body with your arms. Hump your back and gently tuck your head down so you are looking at the front of your thighs. Bracing your arms so you don't bend your elbows, gently raise your head and hollow your back. Repeat slowly 5 times.

20. Leg and Body Hugs

Lie on your back with your knees bent and both feet resting flat on the floor. Bring your left knee up as close to your chest as possible. Grasp it with both hands and gently pull it a little

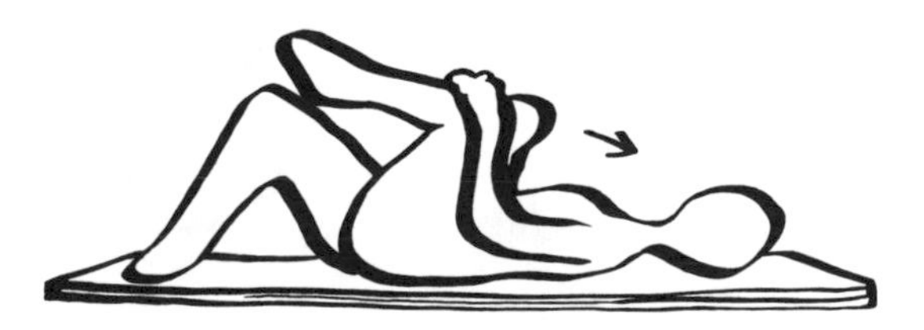

closer to your chest. Hold for a count of 3. Release your knee and slowly lower your leg back down to your original position. Repeat with your right knee. Repeat using both legs for a body hug.

21. Leg Lifts

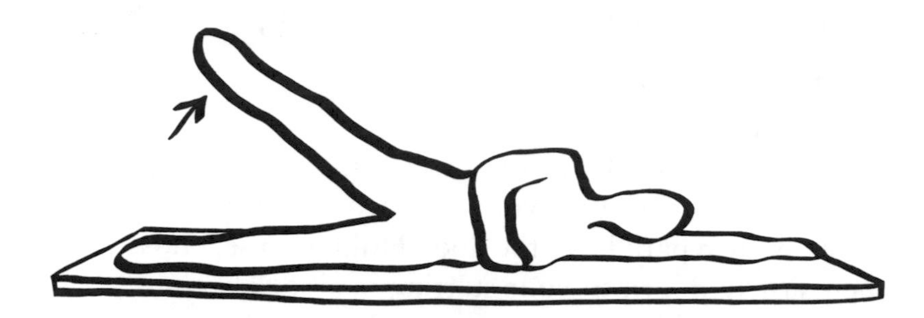

Lie on your left side with both legs straight. With your left arm extended and your head resting on it, use your right arm as support as you raise your right leg slowly to shoulder height in a scissor motion. Repeat 3–5 times. Then bend your right knee and put your right foot on the floor in front of you. Raise your left leg, keeping it straight; point your foot forward. Repeat 3–5 times. Slowly straighten both legs and carefully roll over and repeat on your right side.

22. Inner Thigh Stretch
Sit erect with the bottoms of your feet together. Put your hands on your knees and try to gently push your knees toward the floor. Hold for 5–10 seconds; relax, then repeat.

23. Cross-Legged Side Stretches

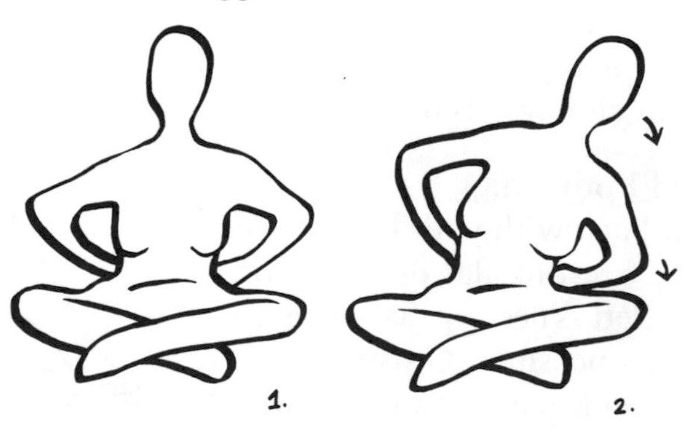

Sit cross-legged with your hands on your hips. Raise your left shoulder and lean to the right, moving your right ear toward your right shoulder. Try to touch your right elbow to the floor. Return to your original position. Repeat on the left side.

24. Thigh Stretches Lying Down
Lie on your left side with your left arm extended and your head resting on it. Bend your right knee and grasp your right ankle with your right hand. Try to bring your right heel back to touch your buttocks. Hold for 15–30 seconds. Roll over and repeat on right side.

ENDURANCE: 15 TO 25 MINUTES

This could be a brisk walk; a jog out of doors; a session on a treadmill, stairmaster or rowing machine; a step or aerobics class; time spent cycling, cross-country skiing or playing tennis; or a combination of the activities below. If you choose indoor activities, you may want to add some lively music that will keep you moving.

1. Marching
Standing tall, march on the spot, raising one knee to waist level, then the other. Swing your arms as you march. To vary the routine, march forward, then backward.

- March forward then backward, punching the air in front of you with your arms at shoulder level.
- March with your arms raised to shoulder level for a count of 10, then lower them down to your sides for a count of 10, and back up again.
- March while moving your arms in a scissor motion, starting with your arms by your sides and your elbows straight. Cross your left wrist over your right wrist, then reverse the movement. As you march, slowly raise your arms to chest level, then move them up to your ear. Lower your arms back to your chest level and then move them down to the low position. Repeat this scissor swing while marching forward and backward.

2. Side Step
Standing tall with your knees slightly bent, step your right foot to the right about 6 inches (15 cm), then bring your left foot over beside it. Repeat. Step to the left and repeat.

3. Jogging
Do gentle jogging if tolerated.

STRENGTH

These are the best bone-building exercises so try to include all of them in your routine.

1. Modified Push-Ups
Lie on your stomach with your palms by your shoulders. Keep your feet together and elevated. Using your arms, raise your upper body while keeping your back straight and your knees touching the floor. Slowly lower your upper body to floor, keeping your feet elevated. Breathe in while pushing up and breathe out as you come down. Start with 5 repetitions and gradually work up to 20.

2. Abdominals: Back-lying
This is a series of exercises to strengthen the lower abdominal muscles. Once you can correctly perform level one, you can progress to the next level and omit the exercise for the previous level(s). Do not progress to the next level until you can move your legs, without your back arching (i.e. your back stays in contact with the floor) for 10 repetitions of the exercise. Remember to breathe.

Level 1

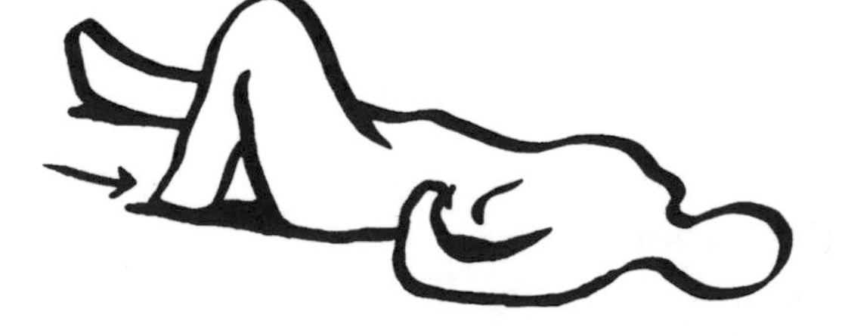

Lie on your back with your legs out straight. Place your fingertips on each side of your abdomen just below your rib cage. Bend your right knee and hip and slowly slide your right heel along the floor, keeping your heel on the floor.

Hold your stomach up and under your rib cage. Slowly slide your heel down, straightening your hip and knee as you return to your starting position. Repeat with the left leg. Repeat 3–5 times, building to 10 times on each side.

Level 2

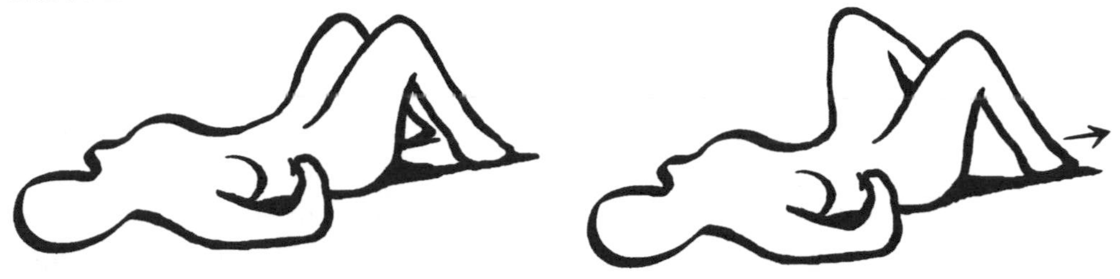

Lie on your back with your hips and knees bent and your feet on the floor. Place your fingertips on each side of your abdomen, just below your rib cage. Bend your right knee as you slowly lift your right foot off the floor, stopping when your thigh is vertical. Repeat with your left leg, while holding your stomach in and keeping your back still. Hold your left leg in this position. Slowly return your right foot to the floor, keeping your knee bent; straighten your leg along the floor. Then slide your left foot back to the starting position. Remember to keep both your pelvis and your back flat on the floor while moving your leg. Repeat 3–5 times, building to 10 times.

Level 3

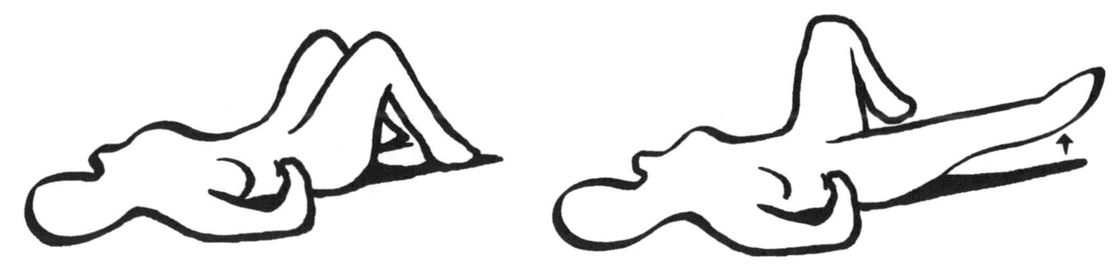

Lie on your back with your hips and knees bent and your feet on the floor. Place your fingertips on each side of your abdomen, just below your rib cage.

Bring both of your knees toward your chest; stop when your thighs are vertical and hips are at 90 degrees. Hold your left leg in this position; straighten your right leg parallel to the floor and slowly lower it to the floor. Return your right leg to the starting position. Then straighten your left leg and slowly lower it to the floor. Keep your abdomen flat and both your pelvis and your back still. Repeat 3–5 times, building to 10 times.

Level 4
Lie on your back with your legs out straight. Place your fingertips on each side of your abdomen, just below your rib cage. Tighten your lower abdominal muscles to tilt your pelvis and reduce the curve in your back. Slide both feet along the floor, keeping your heels on the floor while bringing both your knees toward your chest. Hold, then slowly slide both legs back to the straight position. During the leg movement, keep your abdomen flat and both your pelvis and your back still. Repeat 3–5 times, building to 10 times.

Level 5

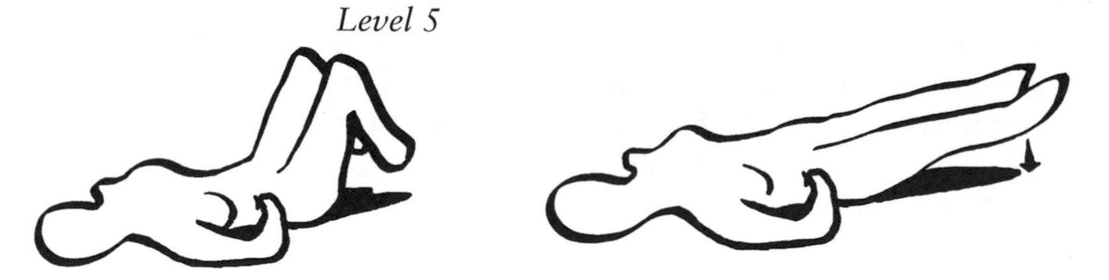

Lie on your back with your legs out straight. Place your fingertips on each side of your abdomen, just below your rib cage.Tighten your lower abdominal muscles to tilt your pelvis and reduce the curve in your back. Bend your knees and hips, bring both feet off the floor and bring your knees toward your chest until thighs are vertical and hips are at 90 degrees. Keeping both heels off the floor, return to the starting position. During the leg movement, keep your abdomen flat and both your pelvis and your back still. Repeat 3–5 times, building to 10 times.

Exercises with Weights

Always follow proper weight-lifting technique:

- These exercises are for fit people. If you have osteoporosis or are at risk for fracture, check with your doctor before doing any exercise program.
- Warm up before using weights.
- When using weights, start with a 1 lb (.45 kg) Velcro wrist weight and work up to a maximum weight of 2 1/2 lb (1.13 kg). When using ankle weights, start with 1 lb (.45 kg) Velcro ankle weights and work up to 5 lb (2.27 kg) Velcro ankle weights. (Weights with Velcro closings are the easiest to use.)
- Practise proper breathing while using weights. Exhale while lifting (exertion) and inhale during relaxation or while at rest.
- Do the exercises slowly without snapping or locking your joints.
- Start with a comfortable number of repetitions and slowly build to a higher number, adding one repetition at a time. You may also do the repetitions in "sets," for example by doing 2 or 3 sets of 5 repetitions each rather than one set of 10 or 15 as you build up your strength. Rest up to a minute between sets. As you become stronger you can build both the number of repetitions and the number of sets you do. Aim for a maximum of 3 sets of 12 repetitions each.

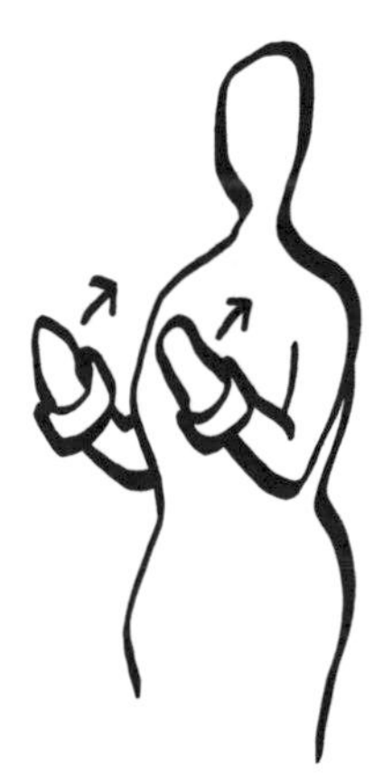

3. Elbow Bends

Standing tall with weights on your wrists and wrists straight, bend your elbows and slowly bring your wrists up to your shoulders and down again. Repeat 3–5 times.

4. Upper Body, Triceps Extensions

Standing tall or sitting with weights on wrist, slowly bring one arm straight up so your elbow is near your ear. Slowly bend your arm, lowering your wrist behind your head. Straighten your arm and repeat 3–5 times, building repetitions. Repeat with your other arm.

5. Heel and Toe Touches

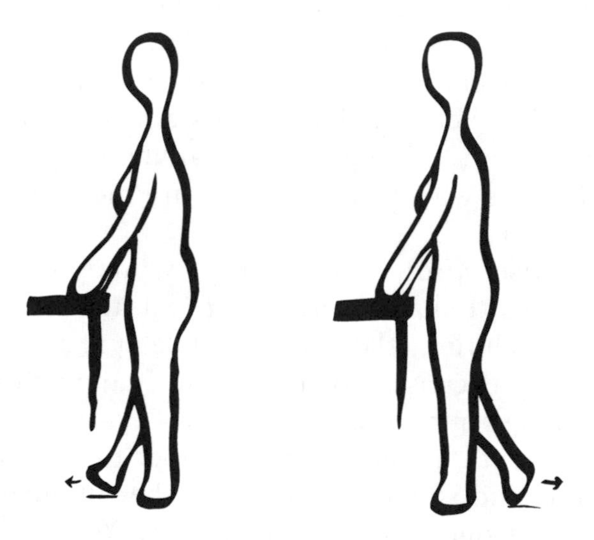

Stand tall with weights on your ankles; hold on to the back of a chair. With your knees slightly flexed, touch the floor in front of you with your right heel, return your right foot to your starting position, and repeat with your left heel. Repeat 10 times. Touch the floor behind you with your right toe, return to your starting position and repeat with your left toe. Repeat 10 times. Build to 3 sets of 10–12 repetitions on each side.

6. Sideways Leg Lift

Stand tall, with weights on your ankle; face a chair back and hold on to it for support. With your toes pointing forward, slowly lift your left leg sideways as far as it will go comfortably. Repeat 3–5 times. Repeat with right leg.

COOL-DOWN: 10 MINUTES

You can use some of the gentle stretching exercises from the warm-up section or try the suggestions below:

1. Slow Dancing
Do any of your favorite steps (such as a waltz) around the room.

2. Stretching Out Against the Wall

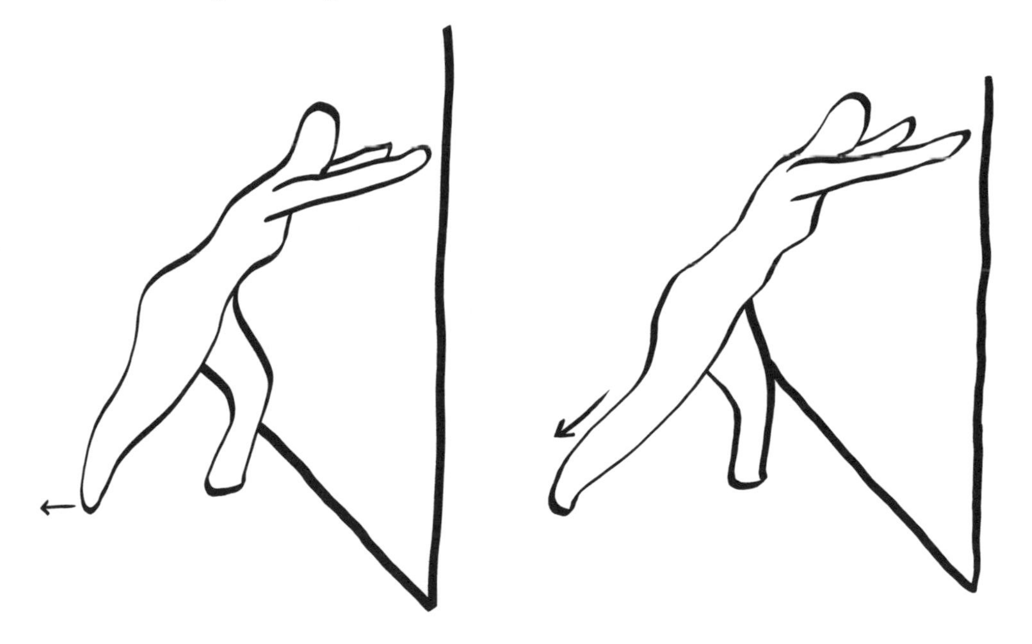

Press your hands against the wall at shoulder height, bend your right knee and slide your left leg straight back as far as it will go while keeping your foot flat on the floor, toes pointing toward wall. Hold the stretch for 15–30 seconds. Repeat with your left knee bent.

3. Hamstring Stretch
Lie on your back, bend your left knee and plant your left foot firmly on the floor. Use your hands to steady yourself as you slowly raise your right leg high over your body to the count of 30. Bring your right leg back down, lift it again to the count of 30 and lower it. Repeat 5 times. Repeat with your left leg.

4. Alphabet Ankle Rotations

Lie on your back, bend your knees and bring one knee up to your chest. Try to write the letters of the alphabet with your foot. Repeat on the other side.

5. Tense and Relax

Lie on your back and tighten all your muscles starting with your toes and moving up to tighten the muscles in your knees and abdomen; squeeze your buttocks together; shrug your shoulders up to your ears and screw up your face. Hold to a count of 5, then relax. Repeat.

6. Relax

Relax into the floor, breathing slowly and deeply. When ready, slowly roll onto your side, bend your knees and slowly push yourself to a sitting position using your hands, then raise yourself to a standing position.

Recipe Index

Subject Index